FITNESS WITHOUT STRESS

A Guide To
The Alexander Technique

by Robert M. Rickover

Published by

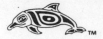

METAMORPHOUS PRESS
P.O. Box 10616
Portland, Oregon 97210

ISBN 0-943920-32-9

Typesetting by Cy-Ann Designs, Portland, Oregon
Printed in U.S.A.

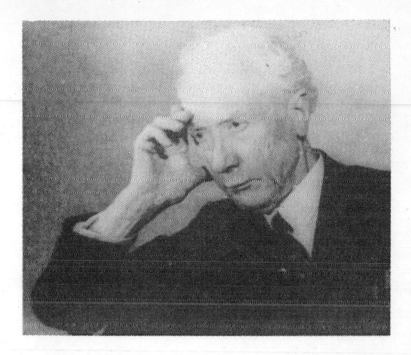

A great deal of the confusion and perplexity in the world today is due to the acceptance and spreading of theoretical concepts which have not sprung from the personal experience of those who advocate them.

F. Matthias Alexander
(1869 – 1955)

ACKNOWLEDGEMENTS

F. Matthias Alexander died in 1955, some twenty years before I was fortunate enough to learn of his work, and the Technique which bears his name. At times I have regretted not having met the man, and experienced his work firsthand. These regrets are shortlived, however, for I have had the privilege of studying with many of the world's finest Alexander teachers.

Among these, I owe a very special debt of gratitude to Marjorie Barstow, Walter Carrington, Eric De Peyer, Patrick McDonald and Peggy Williams, men and women who studied with Alexander and who have devoted their lives to furthering his work. For hundreds of teachers of my generation, they have served as standards of excellence, and as sources of guidance, support and inspiration. I am particularly obliged to Marjorie Barstow and Walter Carrington for taking time from their busy schedules to read the manuscript for this book, and for offering many valuable comments and suggestions.

I would also like to express my appreciation to Elizabeth Rajna Collins, Paul Collins, Margaret Farrar, Vivien Mackie and Susan Thame of the School of Alexander Studies in London, where I received my training. I will always be grateful for their extraordinary skill, dedication and patience. To Kri Ackers, Angela Caine, Elke DeVries, Misha Magidov, Isobel McGilvray, and Olive Scarlett, I extend a special thanks for their valuable help and encouragement during my stay in England.

Among the many pupils, colleagues and friends, whose suggestions and support have been of immense assistance to me in the preparation and the writing of this book, I would especially like to thank Paula E. Valentine, for her generous and skillful editorial assistance, and Edward Maisel for guiding me through the labyrinthine world of book publishing. I would also like to thank Dr. Mel Borins, Jeremy Chance, Peter Cunneen, Michael Frederick, Dr. Joseph Goodman, Emerson Johnson, Verna Johnson, Mitsuki Kikkawa, Dr. Stanley Knebelman, Elaine Kopman, Heather Kroll, Laurie Landy, Frank Ottiwell, Dr. Derek Paul, Jean-Louis Rodrigue, Jonathan and Joanne Rogoff, Kevin Ruddell, Tom Shaw, Steven Slutsky, and Mark Tapia.

I gratefully acknowledge the work of the English author Jane O'Connor Creed who made a substantial and invaluable contribution to the writing of this book.

TABLE OF CONTENTS

FOREWORD

When I first moved my Alexander teaching practice from New York to San Francisco in the mid-sixties, some of the local daily newspapers interviewed me and printed articles about the Technique. I was surprised to see DIFFICULT TO EXPLAIN heading the first article that appeared. I was further chagrined to find under my picture accompanying the article my name, and again the dread phrase "Difficult to Explain" — blessedly in lower case this time.

Describing the Alexander Technique with words alone has been a problem from the beginning. The reality is that true understanding of the Technique comes only with experiencing it, not from reading or talking about it. Still, it is incumbent upon those of us who want more people to experience the benefits of Alexander's work to write and talk about it too.

Since the early 1970s, there has been a phenomenal growth of interest in the Technique. The number of qualified teachers and teacher training courses has increased dramatically and far more material about Alexander's work is now available in print. When I was training to teach in the mid-fifties, there were to my knowledge only five books published on the Technique. Four of those were by F. Matthias Alexander himself and the other one was *Inside Yourself* by Louise Morgan. Louise Morgan's book was written for "popular" (as opposed to serious) consumption and as such was received with some disdain by those surrounding Alexander. Alexander, however, is reported to have said "That book will probably bring more people to the work than my books will."

In writing *Fitness Without Stress — A Guide To The Alexander Technique*, Robert Rickover has deftly combined the popular and the serious. Popular in this case means easily accessible information written in an easy-to-read style, and serious means that the information is solid and well-researched.

The book is a guide — a guided tour, if you like — from the beginning years of the Technique to its present, with a look into its possible future, a guide through the workings of a lesson, and a resource book for those who want to find an Alexander teacher.

As the world of the Alexander Technique continues its rapid expansion, the need for a book of this kind has become evident. Fortunately for all of us, Robert Rickover has taken the time to write it.

Frank Ottiwell, Director
The Alexander Training Institute of
San Francisco

THE FITNESS MYTH

Initial Questions

Several years ago I watched a man kill himself in the name of fitness. I was living on Manhattan's lower West Side at the time and, morning and evening, I couldn't fail to notice the gruelling exercise program of one of my neighbors. Throughout nine months of a bone-chilling New York winter, a regenerating spring and a hot, sultry summer, he jogged through city streets, congested with people, cars and pollutants. I heard from his wife that he had suffered a mild heart attack two years before, and after recovering decided to exercise regularly. He had read somewhere that jogging would keep him fit.

What fascinated me most about his exercise regimen was how uncomfortable he looked. Almost running, rather than jogging, his movements had a frantic and desperate quality to them. His head was pulled tightly back on his neck and his shoulders were raised, as though he carried an enormous burden. His fists were clenched rigidly at each side, and he always wore a painful expression on his face.

It was one morning during the second winter of his program that he collapsed while jogging and died in an ambulance on the way to the hospital — he had suffered a massive coronary.

After what had happened to my neighbor, I was particularly struck a few weeks later by an item in the local community paper. A middle-aged fitness buff, who was a regular at the neighborhood gym, had begun shoveling his car out of a snowdrift. Ten minutes later he was dead of a heart attack.

Why, I wondered, had these two men, who apparently were doing all the right things, been betrayed by their bodies? This is the kind of question which today is being voiced with increasing frequency. Cases proliferate of exercise leading to injury — and even death — instead of health and well being. More and more fitness participants are asking if there are safe — and *un*safe — ways to get fit.

Medical science now understands all too well the possible causes for the two deaths just mentioned. The recent fitness boom has provided the raw material for numerous investigations into the effects of a large or sudden increase in the level of physical activity. These studies have cast very serious doubt on the notion that exercise in any way reduces the likelihood of a stroke or heart attack. What they *have* shown is that the kind of strenuous activities encouraged by many of today's fitness programs can be damaging to our health in a distressing variety of ways, one of which is the aggravation of an existing heart condition.

Fitness and Fashion

Only a total recluse could have failed to notice the dramatic rise in fitness consciousness that has taken place in recent years. Articles on every aspect of this phenomenon appear regularly in the press. Fitness is a feature of countless television programs, along with ads selling us the latest scientifically designed exercise equipment. Bookstores offer workout books and tapes, endorsed by popular movie stars, each one promoting its own special brand of fitness. Business is booming at fitness centers, while having your own personal trainer has become the latest status symbol.

A whole new fashion industry has been created to profit from the manufacture of exercise outfits and accessories. Cosmetic companies have come up with new lines of sweat-proof make-up. The market is flooded with gadgets that check pulse rates, record miles and time exercises. Phrases like "runner's high", "no pain, no gain" and "aerobic burnout" have come into common usage.

For people like me, who grew up in North America in the 1940's and 1950's, today's emphasis on fitness came as quite a surprise. In those days, most people *hated* exercising. By the time we got to high school, my friends and I spent far more time in a car than on our feet. Our interest in athletics consisted mainly of watching baseball on television and turning out to support our school's football and basketball teams.

Newspapers and magazines carried dire warnings that the Russians and Europeans were more fit than us and that we had better shape up. Schools and colleges were encouraged to expand their physical education programs and publicity campaigns sprang up to warn us of the dangers of inactivity.

Who Benefits?

How times have changed! Today, fitness has become a major industry and we are now confronted with a bewildering array of programs. They have become as common as fad diets and street-wise consumers are beginning to ask similar questions: Why are there so many "foolproof" systems, with each one different from the others? Why do such large numbers of people drop out of these programs? Why are so many *forced* to stop because they have seriously injured themselves?

The trend towards keeping fit has been creating a wide range of problems, from the relatively minor inconvenience of a pulled muscle, to more serious injuries like tennis elbow and runner's knee and even permanent handicaps caused by strokes and heart attacks. As hospitals and sports injury clinics struggle to mend the injured, we hear fewer success stories and more tales of disappointment and woe.

The media have treated the public to glimpses of the problem. Television shots of former United States President Jimmy Carter's near collapse while jogging, with his physician helping him to a car, grabbed everyone's attention. The death, while running, of Jim Fixx, author of *The Complete Book of Running* was widely reported in the press. Newspaper headlines are starting to ask, "Are Health Clubs Risky?", "How Fit Is Your Fitness Instructor?", and "Is Exercise Harmful To Your Health?"

The medical community has taken the lead in challenging the assumptions underlying current fitness trends. Too much, or the wrong kind of exercise has been linked to an ever widening variety of health problems. Researchers have even found that over-strenuous activity can weaken our immune system's ability to resist infection and disease.

Henry A. Solomon, M.D., an eminent cardiologist and author of *The Exercise Myth*, a thoughtful survey of today's exercise scene, states succinctly, "Exercise will not make you healthy. It will not make you live longer. *Fitness and health are not the same thing.*" (emphasis mine).

What Is Fitness?

Fitness and health not the same thing? Clearly it's time to take a fresh look at the whole idea of what we really mean by fitness. The word has obviously taken on a new, distorted meaning in recent years. Much the same happened with "health food". Remember when it meant food that was especially nourishing or free from chemicals? Nowadays, the health conscious shopper has to be careful he's not buying ordinary food that's simply been re-packaged in a fancy box with sheaves of grain or an old-fashioned farmhouse pictured on the front.

Originally, "fitness" had a clear and straightforward meaning. The Oxford Dictionary says "fit" means: "to be in harmony with" and "well adjusted or suited for some purpose or status". Webster's New American Dictionary defines "fit" as "put into a condition of readiness".

These are definitions that make a lot of sense and agree with our ordinary understanding of the word. But many of us have been deceived into confusing fitness with such things as weight loss and muscle development.

By itself, deliberately changing one's size or shape is really an attempt to gain the *appearance* of good health. Though it produces a poor substitute for the genuinely pleasing appearance of a well-toned, poised and coordina-ted body, people have sometimes been convinced that merely by losing weight or becoming more muscular they will also become more desirable.

As Dr. Alexander Lowen, M.D., the developer of bio-energetics, laments:

> "For too many people the goal of exercise pro-grams is to *look* (not feel) good, in accord with the current fashion ideal. They want a lean, tight, hard body, capable of performing with machine-like effi-ciency at the command of the will. Or they may aim for a statuesque quality, for the body of a young Adonis or Venus. . . . heavy musculature may make one look strong, but it reduces the body's spontaneity and aliveness and seriously restricts breathing."

Being able to squeeze into a smaller bikini or fill out a

skin-tight t-shirt — which is what so often passes for fitness today — may really reflect a desire for friends, love or success, goals we all share. But attending a *fitness* class to find romance or make business contacts could be a costly mistake. With the real emphasis shifted elsewhere, the fitness program itself is likely to be carried out in a way that ignores your individual needs and capabilities and greatly increases the likelihood of injury or other harmful results.

In an attempt to create the perfect body, "fitness" enthusiasts may even develop eating disorders like anorexia nervosa, or over-enlarge their muscles to the point where performance of day-to-day activities is hindered. Some programs actually encourage this kind of obsessive behavior.

In just a generation, we have gone from a lifestyle which attached little importance to physical training to one which has made fitness a national obsession. In the process, many of the undeniable benefits, and the *fun*, of vigorous physical activity have been lost.

The Heart of the Matter

Increased cardiovascular capacity, another popular fitness goal, *is* very significant. Cardiovascular capacity is a measure of our ability to absorb oxygen, get it to different parts of the body and convert it, along with food, into energy. The rate at which the body can do this is limited by breathing capacity, circulation, condition of the heart and so on.

In the late 1950's and early 1960's, a U.S. Air Force doctor named Kenneth H. Cooper conducted exhaustive tests on airmen to learn more about this important measure. He discovered that it is possible to actually increase our capacity to absorb oxygen. To do this requires exercise which significantly elevates the pulse rate for an appreciable period of time.

As cardiovascular capacity expands, so too does the ability to exercise vigorously for even longer periods. Ordinary walking won't do it. More strenuous exercises like jogging, swimming, squash and cycling will. Dr. Cooper eventually went on to develop a whole set of aerobic exercise regimens designed to systematically expand cardiovascular capacity — and thereby our ability to exercise still more.

Because of its tremendous influence on our thinking about physical fitness, it is easy to forget that today's emphasis on aerobics is a very recent development.

An Incomplete Picture

Dr. Cooper's pioneering work, and his widely-read books, alerted millions to the need for more physical activity in their lives. And he made a major contribution to our understanding of how our body functions.

But, as so often happens with new discoveries, the aerobic conditioning processes he developed have not always been wisely used. The heavy commercial promotion of fitness has encouraged us to forget that aerobic capacity, with its almost exclusive emphasis on the operation of the cardiovascular system, is really just *one* of many important fitness indicators.

Your body is, after all, composed of a lot more than a heart and lungs. You have a head, a neck, shoulders, a spine, hips, legs, ankles, feet and so on. *All* these parts must operate in a coordinated, integrated manner if you are to live your life in an effective and enjoyable way. Being able to pass an aerobics test doesn't in any way guarantee that you will go through life without pain, discomfort and fatigue.

Think about what's involved in a normal day. You probably spend a good deal of time at work. In addition you may also have to clean the house, mow the lawn, shop, attend meetings and take care of the thousand and one other tasks involved in living. If you're in good health, you may well take part in sports or other forms of vigorous activity. And of course you spend time socializing with family and friends.

What most of us really need in the way of fitness is the ability to carry out these daily activities in an enjoyable, easy, efficient manner. We also want the ability to cope with unanticipated crises calmly and effectively. And, finally, we need to be able to get a good night's sleep so that we can awake refreshed and alert the next morning.

Fitness Flaws and Failures

Exercise, as performed in most fitness programs, contributes little to these basic goals. It does nothing to improve the *way* we use our bodies. In fact, it often encourages an exaggeration of our worst habits. You can observe this for yourself the next time you watch a group of joggers or participants in an aerobics class. You can see that many of them look awkward and uncomfortable in their movements. Some may even resemble my jogging neighbor.

Of course it *is* important to take care of our heart and lungs. The more efficiently we convert air and food into energy, the less stress we place on these vital organs. But to develop them at the expense of the rest of the body is doing ourselves a great disservice. As Gilbert Gleim, a physiologist at Manhattan's Lenox Hill Hospital notes, "A strong cardiovascular system doesn't do much good when the other parts of the body are weak or inflexible."

Aerobic capacity is simply a measure of *one* — admittedly significant — aspect of fitness. Unfortunately, it is now often made an end in itself. This has seriously restricted our notion of what fitness is all about, causing us to ignore the many other equally important determinants of good health.

This extremely narrow approach to fitness encourages us to isolate it from other activities, to somehow squeeze it into a busy schedule. Keeping fit can then easily become an activity which isn't enjoyable and which has little carryover or connection to the rest of our lives.

Indeed, many fitness programs treat the body as though it were a machine which should perform on cue, at will. This attitude smothers our natural self-awareness by encouraging us to ignore aches, pains and the many other signals our body uses to let us know when something is wrong. In aerobics classes, loud music, the beat often forcing the rhythm of the exercises, still further desensitizes participants.

The problem is made worse by the unhealthy attitude many fitness instructors take toward their *own* bodies. They may deny, even to themselves, that their back hurts, that they have shin splints, or that their mind has gone numb from listening to hour after hour of loud music. Indeed, it's not uncommon for instructors with serious injuries to continue with a full teaching load. "Aerobics instructors are driven people", observes Dr. James Garrick, Director of the Center for Sports Medicine at Saint Francis Hospital in San Francisco. "And driven people are best at ignoring problems."

Lack of body awareness is clearly a major contributor to the dramatic increase in exercise-related injuries. During an aerobic workout the leg joints, to take just one example, are subjected to an extraordinary amount of stress. Every time a participant's foot pounds onto the ground, three to eight times the body weight can smash onto his or her ankle and knee.

When pain signals are *not* heeded, serious injuries can easily develop. Tendonitis, shin splints, knee problems and fractures are often the unwanted rewards for embarking on a fitness program without having a clear understanding of what fitness is really all about.

The Darker Side of Fitness

The Physicians and Sports Medicine, a medical journal which has been around since 1973, devotes a large portion of its pages to articles about fitness-related injuries and the harmful effects of fitness programs. A selection of titles makes alarming reading: "Sudden Death and Jogging", "Aerobic Dance Injuries — A Symposium", "Knee Disorders in Runners", "Are We Running From the Truth About Exercise?", and "Burnout in Adolescent Athletes".

Fitness instructors themselves are finally beginning to speak out. In a recent radio interview, an experienced instructor, who wished to remain anonymous for fear of losing her job, spoke of seeing her colleagues leading participants down the path to injury:

> "It's a delicate situation because you're mixing business with health standards. I've often seen instructors leading groups that are way too big. One person can't really keep track of a hundred people and make sure they aren't harming themselves. I've seen people doing exercises that are harmful to their back, their legs, their knees. A lot of instructors teach classes with arched backs — like you see on T.V. It may be sexy looking, but it can be *very* dangerous."

Anna, a twenty year old university student, is a typical aerobic dance victim. As a result of severe shin splints, she now must undergo months of unpleasant and painful physiotherapy. Anna says,

"I got shin splints from doing aerobic exercise. Now I have to see the physio-therapist three times a week. I can't do any aerobics now. I can't run. I can't even walk the short distance between classes because my legs hurt so much. The doctor told me not to go back. He said the worst way to get shin splints was through aerobic classes. I wish I'd heard that before."

Quality vs. Quantity

Within the fitness industry a reform movement seems to be underway. Softer floors are being installed, information on injuries is being made available and standards for instructors are being established, reducing some of the most obvious dangers of fitness activities. Unfortunately none of these steps addresses the basic problem.

What we really need is a completely different approach to fitness, one which shifts the emphasis away from today's almost total preoccupation with the *quantity* of exertion. It isn't only the number of miles run, the time spent doing aerobic exercises, or the heaviness of the weights lifted that matters. Far more important is the *quality* of our movements — our balance and coordination and our ease of breathing.

The crucial importance of the way we use our bodies *is* beginning to be recognized in other fields. Take, for example, our understanding of back pain. We've known for a long time that, statistically, more than seventy-five per cent of us will suffer serious back pain sometime during our lifetime. But we now also know, as a result of recent scientific investigations, that the way we stand, sit and perform activities — in other words, our *posture* and how we adapt it to changing circumstances — has a major impact on the amount and kind of pressure we put on our spinal

column and, consequently, on our *personal* chances of becoming a back pain sufferer.

After an exhaustive survey of the evidence amassed in
recent years, Judylaine Fine, Executive Vice President of
The Back Association of Canada and author of *Conquer-
ing Back Pain: A Comprehensive Guide,* concluded:

> "As far as I can see, poor posture and move-
> ment patterns are two of the most important, and
> least understood, causes of back pain."

The importance of posture is also now well understood by arthritis researchers. As Dr. Frederic McDuffie,
Medical Director of The Arthritis Foundation, explains:

> "Bad posture can lead to more pain for a per-
> son with arthritis because it puts unnecessary
> stress on joints and muscles. It can also contribute
> to deformities of the hips, ankles, knees and
> spine."

It is increasingly clear that the loss of our natural balance harms us in a variety of ways. Tony Jones, writing for
the "Ultimate Fitness" series in *Esquire* explains:

> ". . . chronic posture imbalances bend and
> stretch our bodies in unhealthy ways. Skeletal
> and muscular symmetry is distorted. Circulation
> may be impaired. Joints and bones bear added
> pressures. Tension pools in muscles that must
> constantly strain against gravity to maintain us
> upright. After a while, we begin to note small
> crookednesses. Instead of true balance, we are
> held in a complicated array of offsetting compen-
> sations. We feel out of sorts, confined, uncomfor-
> table, unable to concentrate, drained of energy."

Fitness Without The Flaws

Skilled athletes and performers have always placed a high value on balance, flexibility, agility and coordination. A growing interest in activities like yoga, Tai Chi and Aikido reflects the general public's recognition of the importance of these qualities. It is now clear that what is needed is a method that will enable us to bring these same qualities into our daily lives — a method that will help us improve the way we use ourselves in *all* of our activities.

Such a method should help us to expand our inherent capabilities in whatever direction we choose. It should be something we can use for the rest of our lives, something which will help us *prevent* injuries — not cause them — and yet still enable us to enjoy vigorous sports and exercise activities. And, of course, it should be something which will improve the way we look and feel.

We can all think of people we know who somehow seem to carry themselves easily, with poise and balance, and whose movements are a pleasure to watch. These same qualities can frequently be observed in young children. Before reaching the age when they start to interfere with their natural movements, children are active in an unself-conscious and graceful manner. They really *enjoy* what they do, whether listening to a good story, learning a new skill or plunging wholeheartedly into an energetic game or contest. Most young children are completely at home in their bodies.

We were all children once. Can we learn how to reclaim these abilities and use them constructively in our adult lives? Is there a way for us to regain our natural body harmony and be fit, once again, in the true sense of the word?

It is the purpose of this book to introduce you to just such a method — and to a number of individuals who have had firsthand experience with it.

(The following personal account, and those which come after the remaining five chapters of this book, were edited from interviews conducted by the author during the summer of 1986 in London, England; Lincoln, Nebraska, USA; and in Toronto, Canada. In some cases, the names of the interviewees have been changed at their request.)

Steven is a microbiologist in his mid-fifties from Stanford, California.

"I work as a virus researcher in a laboratory and spend a lot of time — anywhere from one to four hours a day — looking through a microscope. Around ten years ago, I started suffering really badly from sciatica in my right leg and from back pain that bending over the 'scope was making worse all the time. I had a series of x-rays which showed no structural damage and I saw various orthopedic people, and a chiropractor too, but that didn't help any.

"If you've had constant back pain, you'll know how desperate you get with it, so I consider myself very lucky in that I wound up seeing a doctor who told me "Don't let anybody get near you with a knife. Surgery won't do anything for you." He not only gave me that excellent piece of advice but he also told me a bit about the Alexander Technique — I'd never even heard of it — and suggested that I give it a try. I did so with a combination — I have to admit — of hope and skepticism.

"I felt even more skeptical when, during that first lesson, the teacher spent most of the time getting me to sit down in a chair and get up out of it again, with a bit of walking around in between. However, she explained that she was using these very simple activities to get me to notice some of the things I did when I moved, and to familiarize me with new ways of sitting, standing and walking.

"I didn't actually notice any change after the first lesson, but the teacher conveyed a sense of calmness and confidence — without making any wild promises to solve my problems — so I decided to have some more lessons and see how things went.

"Pretty soon, I noticed definite, steady progress. No overnight miracles, but the back pain that by now I'd had for a couple of years gradually diminished until, by the end of about three months, there was a definite overall improvement. My leg wasn't hurting anywhere near as much, so naturally I was sleeping better and that meant that I was feeling much healthier in general.

"After a few months, I moved to Stanford where there were no teachers back then. But there were several in San Francisco and I started going to one there. He taught mainly in groups which put a lot more responsibility on the participants to watch themselves, to think for themselves. That appealed to me, though I can see the group approach wouldn't suit everybody.

"Anyway, the improvements have continued. With the increased awareness I have of myself, I have a lot less trouble with the microscope. I no longer scrunch myself over it the way I used to. And I'm not so tense while driving — that's certainly a lot easier and less tiring now.

"It's funny because now I notice my colleagues doing exactly the same scrunched up thing that I used to do. And that used to feel perfectly normal to me!

"Another interesting thing I've been noticing in the past few months is that physical stiffness often seems to go together with a certain amount of mental rigidity. I see this a lot at work and I know that was true for me before I began taking lessons.

"You know, when I think back on it, before I began with Alexander lessons, I would spend more time figuring out how to use a new electric blender than I ever devoted to learning how to improve the way my own body

functions.

"*In general, I feel a lot calmer and more easy going and — I know this will sound like a contradiction — but I have a lot more energy. Naturally, I get a tremendous sense of satisfaction at having made so many improvements. I feel very good about it, and about myself.*"

2

DESCRIBING THE INDESCRIBABLE

I first heard about the Alexander Technique through Mary, a co-worker. Mary was a computer programmer who sang with a local group in her spare time. She spent long hours working at her terminal and frequently complained about backaches. One day, at an office meeting, I noticed that she looked brighter, less tired, more relaxed, and I joked that I hadn't heard her complain recently.

After the meeting, Mary told me that several weeks earlier her singing teacher had suggested she take Alexander Technique lessons to improve her voice. An unexpected benefit of the lessons had been the end of her backaches. When I asked her to tell me more about the Technique, she seemed at a loss for words. She could only tell me what it was *not*. It was not bio-feedback, meditation, hypnosis, psychology, manipulation, exercise, yoga, or a host of other therapies. Frustrated, Mary finally threw her hands up in the air, shook her head and told me, "Rob, if you really want to know what it's like, you'll just have to go and take lessons yourself."

The next day she did give me an article to read which contained a quote from Aldous Huxley, the renowned English writer and thinker, and author of *Brave New World*.

In the article Huxley said:

> "The Alexander Technique gives us all things we have been looking for in a system of physical education: relief from strain due to maladjustment, and constant improvement in physical and mental health. We cannot ask for more from any system; nor, if we seriously desire to alter human beings in a desirable direction, can we ask any less."

Huxley was reluctant to define the Technique. He felt that direct, personal experience was necessary for it to be truly understood. Defining it, he argued, would be like trying to describe the color red to someone who is color-blind.

This aroused my curiosity and I soon found several other interesting descriptions of the Alexander Technique. Dr. Wilfred Barlow, M.D., speaking at a meeting of the Royal Society of Medicine in London had this to say:

> "The Alexander Technique, briefly, is a method of showing people how they are misusing their bodies and how they can prevent such misuse, whether it be at rest or during activity."

Frank Pierce Jones, the former director of the Tufts University Institute for Psychological Research, says the Technique

> "... doesn't teach you something to do. It teaches you how to bring more practical intelligence into what you are already doing; how to eliminate stereotyped responses; how to deal with habit and change. It leaves you free to choose your own goal but gives you a better use of yourself while

you work toward it . . . It opens a window onto the little known area between stimulus and response and gives you the self-knowledge you need in order to change the pattern of your response — or, if you choose, not to make it at all."

Following these two rather formal statements, I came across one by Leo Stein, brother of Gertrude, who called the Technique,

". . . the method for keeping your eye on the ball applied to life."

By now it was becoming clear to me that if I wanted to gain a fuller understanding of what the Alexander Technique was all about, I would have to learn something of its history. I soon found myself in the local library, reading about a remarkable series of events that took place nearly a hundred years ago, half way around the world.

It All Began in Australia

Back in the late 19th century in Australia, an exceptionally gifted Shakespearean actor and reciter, F. Matthias Alexander, was enjoying a successful career in the theatre. Unfortunately he had a problem which greatly affected his stage performances. Alexander's friends told him that while performing he sometimes gasped audibly. Moreover, he was increasingly suffering from hoarseness which sometimes led to a partial loss of voice towards the end of a performance.

For an actor, these were serious problems, and they were getting worse all the time. In an attempt to find a cure for his condition, Alexander consulted a number of doctors and vocal coaches. He carefully followed their instructions for treatment. None of the treatments worked.

Finally, one physician advised him to refrain from reciting and to limit the use of his voice for two weeks prior to a performance. As with all the other treatments, Alexander faithfully followed this one as well. On the day of his next recital, he began in fine form. But, halfway through the performance, his voice began to give out. By the end he could hardly speak.

The physician advised him to continue the treatment but Alexander decided that since neither that nor any of the others had been successful, there was no point in continuing. In any case, Alexander was beginning to suspect that his problems were most likely caused by something he was unknowingly doing to himself. After thinking about it, his doctor agreed but was unable to offer any advice or even suggestions as to where Alexander could turn for help. No one, apparently, had ever pursued this line of reasoning before.

Unique Experiments

Alexander began by observing himself with mirrors, both reciting and speaking normally. After doing this for several months, he noticed that he always tightened the muscles in the back of his neck when reciting. This tightening pulled his head back and down onto his spine. At the same time, he constricted the muscles around his throat. The resulting pressure on his vocal chords was the cause of his speech problems.

Once he had made this discovery, the cure was obvious: he simply had to stop tensing the muscles in his neck and throat when he spoke. The cure may have been obvious but it was an entirely different matter when he tried to put it into practice. Each time Alexander thought that he'd succeeded in releasing these muscles, what he saw in the mirrors told him that he was completely mistaken. He was still pulling his head back and down when he started to speak. In fact, the harder he tried to control his body through will-power, the more he unconsciously reverted to his old habits.

Imagine Alexander's frustration. He knew exactly what he wanted to change, but he couldn't get his body to cooperate. He kept falling back into his old habits automatically because they *felt* right. After all, he'd been using his voice in the same way for years. Any attempt to deviate from his long-standing patterns of speech and movement felt completely different — and *wrong*. He finally had to admit that what he experienced as "right" and "wrong" sensations were based on his old habits and were almost completely unreliable guides to the changes he wanted to make.

His long and careful observations in the mirrors also revealed that it wasn't just while speaking that he tightened his neck muscles. This tendency accompanied the start of *all* his actions. And the trouble was not confined to his neck. His whole torso shortened and narrowed as well, interfering significantly with his ability to move and breathe freely. It became clear to Alexander that he could never solve his voice problem without changing habits of which he was largely unconscious but that nonetheless affected his entire body.

Most of us would probably have given up. However, Alexander was determined to get back on stage even though he knew that he would have to throw out all his previous assumptions and start from scratch. And so, during the next years of his life, every spare moment he could find was devoted to performing movement experiments on himself, seeking a way to free himself from the shackles of his habitual, instinctive physical reactions.

Because his body was not responding accurately to his intentions, his primary task was to find a different way to send those mental directions to his body — a way that would prevent his deeply entrenched habits from interfering. It was no easy task. He made many false starts and encountered a good deal of frustration along the way, but eventually his determination and dedication paid off.

After nearly ten years of observation and study, he developed a method of stopping the harmful tensions in his neck and in the rest of his body. His voice problem disappeared and he resumed his career. As an added benefit, he found that he could apply what he had learned to all of his activities, not just acting and reciting. He could now go about his daily tasks with much less tension and a greater degree of ease and economy of effort.

Many years later he wrote a full account of his remarkable odyssey of self-discovery in his third book, *The Use of The Self*.

An Unanticipated Career Change

Alexander's original motive was simply to overcome his own distressing vocal condition and continue his career as an actor. However, when the changes he had made in himself became apparent, friends and fellow actors began asking for help with their own performance problems. Many complained of hampered breathing, speaking difficulties, movement limitations and lack of stamina.

Alexander thought he would be able to explain to them what he had discovered, and what he had done, and that they would then be able to make the same changes themselves. But very quickly he found that simply *telling* them wouldn't work. Their translation of his words into actions frequently produced a result which was the *opposite* of what he meant.

Just as he had earlier been unable to accurately translate his own intentions into movements, many of his early pupils found it difficult to follow his verbal instructions correctly. Alexander concluded that he would also have to *show* them what he had learned. The most direct and effective way to do this, he discovered, was to use his hands to monitor and gently guide the physical responses of his pupils while they listened to his verbal instructions.

Not Just for Entertainers

Alexander came to realize that many of the problems which performers had on stage were due to a tendency to exaggerate their everyday movement habits. In his own case, for example, he tensed his neck and throat muscles a bit *whenever* he spoke. But because of the special demands of reciting in front of a large audience, this harmful habit intensified during performances with, as we have seen, disastrous effects.

You can easily witness this phenomenon for yourself. The next time you turn on the T.V., watch the people who are *not* used to being on camera. Game shows and newscasts, where ordinary people are interviewed, provide many examples. If you look closely you'll begin to notice all sorts of awkward, jerky and inappropriate body movements, for example little twitchings of the arms and shoulders. When people speak, you can often see their necks tense, causing their heads to be pulled backward or to one side — exactly the same sort of habits that plagued Alexander. Sometimes you can actually *hear* the strained quality of their voices and their gasps for breath. With a little practice, you may even be able to spot some of the professionals doing the same kinds of things, though usually more subtly.

As Alexander gained experience in teaching, it became clear to him that the kind of problems he had overcome were really quite common. Of course, they show up differently in each person. But what he observed to be almost universal was a failure to allow the head to balance freely on top of the spine because of excess tension in the muscles of the neck. This produces a downward pull on the spine, the torso, the joints and the limbs and a loss of poise and natural balance in our upright posture. We then lose our once innate ability to function in an easy, efficient manner. This misuse of ourselves can produce a wide variety of unpleasant, often painful, symptoms.

Given the universal scope of the problem, and his early success in helping others, it's not surprising that Alexander became a popular teacher and that the range of his pupils quickly broadened. People started to come for help with problems as diverse as backaches, migraines and insomnia. His teaching method was proving to be an extraordinarily effective way of dissolving long-standing destructive habits, and helping the body to right itself.

An Appreciative Audience

Alexander's work soon came to the attention of local doctors and a number of them began to send patients to him. Among these was Dr. J. W. Stewart McKay, an internationally-known physician and surgeon in Sydney, who encouraged Alexander to take his discoveries to London. McKay believed that it was imperative that Alexander's work be known on a much wider scale.

By the time Alexander left for England in 1904, his experiences had convinced him of these three important truths:

1) Most of us habitually sit, stand, breathe and move about in ways that put a good deal of unnecessary and harmful pressure on our bodies.

2) Because these harmful habits have often been with us for years, in some cases going back even to childhood,

we are generally unaware of them. What we *do* notice is their undesirable effects.

3) It *is* possible to learn to recognize and stop these bad habits and thereby acquire a more graceful and healthier use of ourselves.

In London, Alexander quickly gained wide recognition. Dr. McKay had paved his way with letters of introduction and Alexander's reputation grew quickly, with his first students coming mainly from theatrical circles. Five years after his arrival, the Australian government sent a representative to England to investigate the latest developments in physical education. He reported favorably on Alexander's work and noted that,

> "It is no exaggeration to say that most of the leaders of the dramatic profession in London are enthusiastic believers in the efficacy of (Alexander's) system and many of them have placed themselves under him for tuition."

Sir Henry Irving, the world famous Shakespearean actor, even hired Alexander to wait in the wings during his performances so that he could be helped between acts.

It wasn't long before prominent people in other fields heard about Alexander. One of his first supporters was Professor John Dewey, the great American educational philosopher and reformer. When Dewey first came to Alexander, he was in poor health. His body was very stiff, his breathing shallow and he tired easily. After only a few lessons he noticed a striking improvement, especially with his breathing and his vision. In later years Dewey's doctors frequently commented on his remarkable vitality and good physical condition, particularly the elasticity of his rib cage. Dewey attributed this to the help he had received from Alexander.

As already mentioned, Aldous Huxley was another

supporter. When he began lessons with Alexander, Huxley was so exhausted most of the time that he could only write while lying on his back, typewriter balanced on his chest. The improvements that came from his lessons soon allowed Huxley to write with ease and even speak in public again. Huxley's wife wrote:

> "Alexander has certainly made a new and un-recognizable person of Aldous, not physically only but mentally and therefore morally."

Other well-known people had a lot to say of Alexander and his Technique.

Distinguished American Biologist, Professor George Coghill:

> "Mr. Alexander's method lays hold of the in-dividual as a whole, as a self-vitalizing agent. He reconditions and reeducates the reflex mechanisms and brings their habits into normal relation with the functioning of the organism as a whole."

Sir Stafford Cripps, Chancellor of the Exchequer, the British equivalent of the U.S. Secretary of the Treasury:

> "Instead of feeling one's body to be an aggregation of ill-fitting parts, full of friction and dead weights pulling this way and that so as to render mere existence in itself exhausting, the body becomes a co-ordinated and living whole, composed of well-fitting and truly articulated parts. It is the difference between chaos and order and so between illness and good health."

George Bernard Shaw:

"Alexander established not only the beginnings of a far-reaching science of the involuntary movements . . . but a technique of correction and self control which forms a substantial addition to our very slender resources in personal education."

Indeed the list is long of distinguished and ardent advocates of the Alexander Technique. It includes Sir Charles Sherrington, the great British neurophysiologist and Nobel Prize winner, Professor Nikolaas Tinbergen, ethologist and Nobel Laureate, Professor Raymond Dart, the distinguished anthropologist, and William Temple, Archbishop of Canterbury.

Over the years many members of Britain's medical community have enthusiastically backed Alexander's work and urged other doctors to investigate Alexander's teaching for themselves. As early as 1936, a group of nineteen prominent physicians wrote a letter to the British Medical Journal in which they described the remarkable and consistent improvement in patients they had sent to Alexander, including those suffering from chronic diseases.

Continuous Refinements

Throughout his life, Alexander worked to improve his own teaching skills. During the early years of his teaching, he also trained his brother, Albert Redden Alexander, and a few assistants to help him with his work. But by the 1920's, the need for more trained teachers had become obvious. In 1931 Alexander established a teacher-training course in London and several years later he and his brother began to train teachers in the United States. The very high standards and traditions of these early Alexander schools

— three years of full-time study, small classes and intensive instruction involving first-hand, personal experience with the Alexander Technique — are still practiced today at recognized Alexander teacher training centers.

Alexander was a down-to-earth man whose first concerns were always: "Does it work?" and "Is it beneficial?" In other words: How can you use what you know to improve your life? Alexander had little patience with people who failed to use their knowledge constructively. Once, after meeting with a group of eminent anatomists, he scornfully — and skillfully — mimicked their awkward movement patterns. As far as Alexander was concerned, their vast knowledge of the human body was of little use if they couldn't apply it to their own functioning. Largely self-taught, he believed that it was important to be able to apply knowledge in a practical way.

In 1947, at the age of seventy-nine, Alexander suffered a major stroke which paralyzed the left side of his body. Remarkably, he soon regained substantial use of his arm and leg and within a few months was again giving lessons. Alexander was always one to learn from his own experiences and this proved to be no exception. The stroke had weakened him considerably and he needed to find ways to conserve his energy. His teaching began to take on a more subtle, yet even more powerful form. In the process of regaining his health, he learned ways to further refine his teaching skills.

Alexander taught up until a few days before his death at the age of eighty-six. Photographs and a film clip of him in his last years show an alert, bright-eyed man moving with grace, agility and even playfulness. What better testimony could there be to the effectiveness of his Technique?

Scientific Evidence

John Dewey maintained that, "Mr. Alexander's teaching is scientific in the strictest sense of the word." In his introduction to *The Use of The Self*, Dewey wrote:

"Those who do not identify science with a parade of technical vocabulary will find in this account the essentials of scientific method in any field of inquiry. They will find a record of long, continued, patient, unwearied experimentation and observation in which every inference is extended, tested, corrected by further more searching experiments."

Nonetheless, academic acceptance of the Alexander Technique was hampered for many years by a lack of quantifiable scientific evidence of its effects on pupils. Dr. Frank Pierce Jones, of the Tufts University Institute of Experimental Psychology, was the first investigator to provide the necessary experimental data. Jones' studies, conducted mainly in the 1950's and 1960's, were reported in a number of scientific journals. He used such tools as strobe and action photography, to follow the trajectory of movement and strain gauges, which measure the amount of force exerted in performing actions like sitting, walking, bending, running. In addition, X-rays, electromyography and other modern techniques were used to record the changes which take place during an Alexander lesson. A summary of his studies can be found in his book, *Body Awareness in Action.*

When Professor Nikolaas Tinbergen won the 1973 Nobel Prize for Medicine, he devoted a major portion of his acceptance speech to the Alexander Technique. He reported that he and his entire family had experienced marvelous benefits from lessons. In his speech, reprinted in

Science, Tinbergen said:

> "From personal experience we can already confirm some of the seemingly fantastic claims made by Alexander and his followers, namely, that many types of underperformance and even ailments, both mental and physical, can be alleviated, sometimes to a surprising extent, by teaching the body musculature to function differently. . . . . We already notice, with growing amazement, very striking improvements in such diverse things as high blood pressure, breathing, depth of sleep, overall cheerfulness and mental alertness, resilience against outside pressures, and also in such a refined skill as playing a stringed instrument."

More recently, research at Columbia Presbyterian Medical Center in New York has shown that lessons in the Alexander Technique can produce a significant increase in breathing capacity — a key indicator of our level of cardiovascular fitness.

It seems fitting that some of the most exciting new scientific research on the Technique is now underway in Australia. Dr. David Garlick, Senior Lecturer in the School of Physiology and Pharmacology at the University of New South Wales, is currently using sophisticated recording and computing equipment in conducting a detailed study of the mechanisms underlying Alexander's discoveries.

An Evolution

Pupils of the Alexander Technique have always been mainly attracted by the concrete, practical benefits of their lessons — benefits that can indeed be quite dramatic. But Alexander also made some profound and fundamental contributions to our understanding of the process by which our mental directions are transformed into physical actions. It is no exaggeration to say that over the course of his lifetime he singlehandedly laid the foundations for a revolutionary new science of human movement, the implications of which are only now beginning to be fully appreciated.

Alexander's thinking was always far ahead of his time. It is, after all, only in the last twenty years or so that the intimate connection between mind and body has become widely accepted in Western medical and scientific circles. Certainly in the 1890's, when Alexander was conducting his initial experiments, this notion was considered eccentric and bizarre. Even now, the importance he attached to the manner in which we use our bodies is a comparatively novel idea.

During the many years of his meticulous observations and rigorous testing of his theories — first working on himself and later helping others — Alexander made a number of very important discoveries about human behavior. While most of the rest of this book is devoted to the practical aspects of the Technique, in the Epilogue we will explore some of the broader issues raised by his discoveries.

At the time of Alexander's death, in 1955, the Technique was well known only in the United Kingdom and in a few cities in North America. Because of the need for intensive individual training, teachers cannot be mass-produced. Moreover, the training process was severely disrupted by World War II when most teachers entered military service. Consequently the number of teachers grew quite slowly for many years. If you had heard of the Alexander Technique as recently as fifteen or twenty years ago, you might have had to travel a thousand miles to find a teacher.

In the years since Alexander's death, and particularly in the last decade, the Alexander Technique has won recognition on a much broader scale. The United States, Europe, Israel, Canada, and Australia all have increasing numbers of Alexander teachers. More and more doctors, dentists, chiropractors and other health-care professionals are aware of its benefits and regularly refer patients for lessons. Governments are funding programs for both teacher training and rehabilitation work. Most of the world's most prestigious schools for actors, singers and musicians include courses in the Alexander Technique.

Among the general public, there's been a dramatic upsurge of interest in the Technique. Several books and innumerable articles on the subject have appeared in America, Britain and other countries. The Technique has also been featured in radio and television broadcasts on both sides of the Atlantic.

One thing, however, has remained the same: the difficulty of giving a clear definition of the Technique. In many other areas of our lives, we are familiar with the problem of trying to express in words our non-verbal feelings and experiences. The Alexander Technique is no exception. When I am pressed to provide a definition, I always emphasize the *process* which lies at the heart of the Technique: learning how to look at ourselves objectively; recognizing habits which are responsible for pain or discomfort, or which interfere with our ability to carry out activities; determining the best way to change those habits; and then setting about changing them. That's the sequence Alexander went through to solve his own voice problem, and it's precisely what present day pupils of the Technique learn to do — with indispensable guidance from a trained teacher.

A Solution

We know that our physical condition affects our health and the quality of our lives. The tremendous interest in fitness expresses this understanding. At the same time, we are wise to be apprehensive about embarking on a fitness program which may do us more harm than good.

The Alexander Technique plays a unique and important role here. What pupils learn during Alexander lessons can be applied to any situation. Knowing how to eliminate unnecessary tension and harmful movement patterns can bring a far greater degree of safety and effectiveness to sports and other vigorous physical activities. Even ordinary everyday activities can be carried out with greater ease, efficiency and enjoyment.

In the following chapter, we will take a look at some of the specific ways the Alexander Technique can help *you*.

Rosalind, who is in her early thirties, is a riding teacher and the co-owner of a riding school in Dorset.

"I was first introduced to the Alexander Technique by the mother of one of my pupils. She gave me a pamphlet on the application of the Alexander Technique to riding. The author started by talking about his back problem that had been helped by the Technique. This immediately grabbed my attention and my interest because at the time I was having a lot of trouble with my back as a result of an accident four years previously. I'd been helping to hitch a horse trailer onto a car. It slipped and when I tried to lift it, I damaged my back.

"I'd seen an orthopedic surgeon, an osteopath, even a masseuse, but while there were brief remissions, basically the trouble never went away. None of the help I got was anything other than temporary. I'd get sore from riding one day, that soreness would get worse the next, and finally it would get so bad that I couldn't ride and I'd just have to take a couple of weeks off. Although I hated the thought

of it, I was having to consider the possibility of changing my career — it's no good having a riding teacher that can't ride!

"After reading the pamphlet, I located an Alexander teacher in a neighboring market town and went for a private lesson. She started working with me on a table and I distinctly remember getting off the table with a real feeling of lightness and no pain. This was quite remarkable and, naturally, I continued with the lessons. There hasn't been any time since then that I haven't been able to ride — my back gets a bit sore now and then, but nothing like before.

"The lessons have also had all sorts of other, quite unexpected effects. First and foremost of these is the way the Technique has influenced my teaching. After a few Alexander lessons, I realized that everything I said to my riding pupils was affecting the way they used their bodies. For the first time, I could see that they were using themselves in ways that were pretty damaging to themselves and to the horses. Once I had understood this, I had to fundamentally rethink the way I taught, the kind of instructions I gave — even the tone of the instructions and the general atmosphere of the lesson.

"I started to think — and talk — much more in terms of soft, resilient bodies flowing with the horse's movement and energy — instead of hard, pushing bodies trying to force movement out of the horse. And this new approach was remarkably successful. It's a way of getting the horse to do what you want him to do without a lot of strain and force — like an extension of how you are using the Alexander Technique in relation to your own body and physical actions.

"In fact, now I come to think of it, there are striking parallels between the worst aspects of some riding approaches and the way we misuse our own bodies. What I mean is that, in riding, a lot has come down through the military style of thinking — the assumption that if you

push and pull hard enough you can get the result you want. You can dominate the animal. Whereas if you learn to recognize the ways the horse needs to move, and encourage his own easy use, you get a much better performance. Traditionally, we push the horse and make him uncomfortable and make him want to run forward. This way, you just make it easy for the horse to do what you want him to do. He's contented instead of harassed and he'll respond much more accurately to your intentions.

"If I had to sum up what the Alexander Technique has done for me, I think I'd say that it has taught me, in all sorts of ways, to go with the flow. And I certainly don't mean that in a weak-willed, fatalistic way — I have no patience with that kind of thing. I mean in the sense of doing everything, as far as possible, in the most natural way possible — which turns out — I must admit to my own surprise, rather — to be also the easiest and the most effective."

3

HOW THE ALEXANDER TECHNIQUE CAN HELP YOU

Why Take Lessons?

As we saw in the last chapter, some of the most distinguished thinkers of his time — among them John Dewey, Aldous Huxley and George Bernard Shaw — drew attention to F. M. Alexander's work and publicly discussed the impact he had on the development of their intellectual and philosophical ideas. However, right from the start of his teaching, it was mainly for practical reasons that people came to him. They wanted relief from unpleasant physical sensations or an improvement in their performance skills — sometimes both — and his reputation steadily grew with his successes in these areas.

A great many people still go to Alexander teachers for these same reasons. Often, it is to end the pain caused by backaches, migraines, stiff necks and the like. Or they want a way to overcome performance-related difficulties. A singer having trouble with her breathing and a violinist whose bowing arm has become stiff are two very common examples. But, what pupils soon notice — often with surprise and even skepticism at first — is that the Alexander teacher does not immediately focus on their specific difficulties. On the contrary, the teacher's primary concern is with the way the pupil uses his or her entire mind/body "mechanism".

For this reason, no matter what has caused the pupil to come to an Alexander teacher, the first few lessons almost always start with ordinary activities such as sitting down in a chair, standing up or walking. These things, which we all do many times every day, provide a useful framework within which the teacher can familiarize the pupil with his movement habits — helping him to recognize, and then prevent, the ones that are harmful.

A Man "Before His Time"

This approach was always part and parcel of Alexander's own teaching. He emphasized, over and over again, that the only effective way to get rid of unwanted symptoms was to recognize and change the interconnected set of harmful posture and movement habit patterns that was at the root of the problem. All his experience had shown him that it made no sense to treat one part of the body as though it were separated from the rest or to treat it without considering repercussions elsewhere.

Nor did it make sense to think in terms of "mind" and "body" as two entirely distinct entities. In his books, he often used the term *psychophysical* as a way of emphasizing the complete involvement of all aspects of ourselves in whatever we do. "Nature does not work in parts," he once wrote. "She treats everything as a whole."

In other words, at least half a century before "wholistic" became a concept familiar to all of us, Alexander was teaching precisely that approach to physical well-being.

Good Use — Bad Use

Alexander's work with himself, and his early pupils, clearly showed that the way we use our bodies determines how well we function. With *good use* (a phrase borrowed by Alexander from the language of horsemen) movements are graceful, pleasurable and coordinated — a joy to watch. There is no unnecessary pressure or tension placed on the body. Our bodies are balanced, poised, ready to do whatever we want, whenever we want to do it.

Mis-use produces movements that are tense and awkward, postural positions that are rigidly held. For example, shoulders may be pulled forward and down onto the chest, or perhaps the opposite — held tightly back, almost in a military manner. *Any* holding or fixing of postural positions harms our coordination and our ability to carry our intentions into action.

Mis-using your body can be compared to driving a car at high speed in low gear with poorly aligned wheels, and defective brakes. You'll probably still get to your destination. But it takes a great deal more energy than is really necessary, exposes you to unnecessary danger, and produces a lot of harmful wear and tear.

If you would like to see some examples of good use in your own environment, watch the movements of a domestic cat, or of small children as they walk, run, play and sit. Both have an alive, in-the-moment quality, giving themselves over entirely and easily to every movement they make.

Alexander himself especially loved watching acrobats. He went to the circus to do so whenever he could because their skill in movement beautifully represented what he was aiming for in his own teaching.

As a boy, when my parents took me to the circus, I remember being impressed by the acrobats' children as they practiced tightrope-walking on the guy wires of the

tents. Some of them no doubt went on to become performers themselves. Of course, they were in the best possible
place to learn the specific skills they would need. But an
even greater advantage was their constant exposure to the
very high standards of coordination and balance of their
parents and of the other circus people. Most of these kids
grew up without ever losing the basic abilities needed for a
successful career in the circus.

People in other occupations which require exceptional
physical skills frequently show this same alertness, balance
and economy of effort. Fred Astaire, and Muhammad Ali
in his prime, are two well-known examples.

Habits: Help or Hindrance?

You and I may not want to walk a high wire or do
daring trapeze acts but we would like to move with ease
and efficiency as we go about our day-to-day activities.
For example, if your phone now rang, and you got up
from your chair, walked across the room and picked up
the receiver, you would, without thinking much about it,
probably have carried out a complex set of movements in
an automatic, habitual way. We rely on the habits we have
developed in order to live efficiently. If we had to think
about every movement we made, life would become very
complicated — and boring!

The problem is that some of our habits are *not* helping
us. In fact, they can even be quite harmful. Moreover, as
these habits may be subtle ones, we can be totally unaware
of them, despite the fact that they may be creating severe
physical problems. That was the first obstacle Alexander
himself had to overcome when he began his experiments.
He didn't know how he mis-used himself because the ways
in which he moved and spoke seemed normal to *him* —
they were what he'd always done.

However oblivious we might be to our harmful movement habits, we are certainly aware of their effects. We
may get backaches, headaches, perhaps feel un-coordinated
or are easily tired. We may find it painful to do ordinary
activities like climbing a flight of stairs. These unpleasant
sensations are the only ways left for our body to tell us
we're doing something wrong.

To solve his own problem, Alexander had to start
thinking about his movements — *and* his thinking itself —
in a whole new way. Even when he got to the point where
he could clearly see his bad habits in the mirrors, he
couldn't get rid of them by a simple act of will. He had to
re-learn, with an almost childlike ability, to stay in the moment as his conscious thoughts directed his movements; he
had to forge a clear link between what he *wanted* to do
and what he *actually* ended up doing. It is precisely this
skill which pupils learn today — "thinking in activity", a
phrase John Dewey used to describe the Alexander process.

There are a great many specific areas in which this process can be applied. Let's take a look at a few of them,
along with some of the benefits pupils have derived from
their lessons in the Alexander Technique.

Backache

The Alexander Technique has a long history of helping
people with back pain. This is not surprising as patterns of
muscular mis-use and mal-coordination can subject the
spinal column to extremely damaging twists and pressures.
These abnormal forces frequently produce structural distortions, such as an undue compression, or exaggerated
curvature of the spine. Even a mild deformity of this kind
adversely affects the way the entire body weight is carried,
and so can often be the cause of severe pain in the back or
elsewhere in the body.

Typically, some back muscles have become constantly over.contracted, while others remain unduly slack. Because this takes place on a continuous basis, day after day, year after year, we are often completely unaware of what's going on until a painful symptom like backache appears — suddenly and without warning, often in middle age.

Pupils sometimes wonder how they could have been tightening their back muscles so severely without knowing it. I ask them to clench one fist, as tightly as possible. Of course, they feel the tension, but, after a few minutes, the sensation starts to diminish. If they were to continue for a day or so, they probably wouldn't feel a thing. They might even forget that they had a hand!

The human body works with great efficiency. Initially it sends repeated messages to the brain, "Hey, something's wrong here." But if those messages are ignored long enough, the body simply stops wasting the energy required to send them. And so the tension can continue, unnoticed, until pressures build to a crisis point.

Undoing this harmful pattern requires a *release* of over-contracted muscles, as well as an improvement in the tone of others. Unfortunately, the "muscle-strengthening" exercises given to backache sufferers often make matters worse because they require contraction, or shortening, of the very muscles that are already much too tight. Instead of making these muscles stronger, as intended, this additional contraction actually *weakens* still further their ability to support and move the body.

Indeed, almost all exercises tend to build up musculature on the basis of distortions that are already present. It's really very much like the proverbial crooked man who walked a crooked mile. A sway-backed man or woman will almost inevitably do a sway-backed exercise. In fact, exercise often causes us to exaggerate our *worst* habits, thus imbedding them even more deeply.

Traction, manipulation, heat treatments, drugs, and

the like, may bring *temporary* relief from the symptoms. But they do little or nothing to overcome the underlying causes. For this, what is necessary is the kind of fundamental, overall, improvement in posture and movement patterns which the Alexander Technique teaches.

Fortunately, there is now a growing recognition of this need in the medical community. Albert W. Grokoest, Clinical Professor of Medicine at the Columbia University College of Physicians and Surgeons, states:

> "Proprioception — muscle, tendon, and joint sense, which has to do with the automatic maintenance of posture and the knowledge of the position of the skeletal musculature of the body — is the basis of the Alexander Technique. It is physiologically logical. No wonder the Technique works so successfully in optimally lengthening tight, in spasm, skeletal muscles."

Dr. Michael G. Neuwirth, Assistant Clinical Professor, Mount Sinai School of Medicine, Associate Chief of the Scoliosis Service at the Hospital for Joint Disease, Orthopaedic Institute, New York, states:

> "As an orthopedist, I have referred patients specifically with postural problems and back and neck pain, who have experienced pain relief after a series of lessons in the Alexander Technique."

Dr. Wilfred Barlow, a British medical specialist in rheumatic diseases and author of *The Alexander Technique* sums it up when he writes:

> "It cannot be emphasized too strongly, so I will write it in capitals. IT IS WRONG TO TREAT A PAINFUL BACK AS A LOCAL CONDITION.

BACK PAIN IS ALWAYS ACCOMPANIED AND
PRECEDED BY GENERAL MIS-USE."

Sleeplessness

Feeling sleepy is simply your body's way of saying,
"I'm tired, I need rest." But our awareness of what our
body is trying to tell us may be blocked by tension and
then we can't fall asleep even when our body needs to re-
cuperate. This same tension also interferes with the natural
muscular relaxation that goes with the changes in breathing and circulation, and all the other physiological adjustments, that are an indispensable part of falling asleep. Of
course the *frustration* of not being able to sleep only adds
to the tension, making the problem even worse.

As we have seen, the Alexander Technique helps pupils
avoid unnecessary tension by teaching them how to become more sensitive to themselves, and how to re-direct
their energies in a more constructive way. Then, when
their body signals that it needs to rest, they are more likely
to feel drowsy, go to bed, *and* fall soundly asleep. After a
good night's sleep, they can awake refreshed, without
having to carry the burden of the past tensions and
anxieties into the new day.

Asthma

An easy flow of air into or out of the lungs is made
possible by the ability of the diaphragm and the rib cage
to move freely. With asthma, the diaphragm tenses and the
ribs fix, prohibiting the lungs from expanding and con-
tracting freely. As the flow of air is restricted, the asth-
matic's instinctive reaction is to become fearful. This fear
may produce additional tension, which restricts breathing

still more. It can all too easily become a vicious circle.

The Alexander Technique teaches asthmatics to stop interfering with what ought to be a very natural process. By helping to release overly contracted muscles, particularly those in the abdomen, lower back, neck, ribs and shoulders, room is provided for all the body's internal organs. The easy rise and fall of the diaphragm and the free expansion and contraction of the ribs makes it possible for the lungs to take in and release air with no unnecessary effort.

Dr. Barlow had this to say concerning the Alexander Technique and breathing disorders in general:

> "There is no shortage of information about the *physiology* of breathing — most of us know that too little oxygen or too much carbon dioxide will make us want more air and we know that various reflex mechanisms in the brain, blood vessels and lungs will work automatically to keep the breathing process going. This is what starts happening when we are born. This is what stops happening when we die. But this physiological account of reflex breathing does not tell us much about *how to breathe*. It is not only in the sphere of medicine that there is that lack of knowledge. Actors, singers, speech teachers, and speech therapists have a special need to know about breathing, as, of course, have all teachers of physical education. Yet in all of these fields — medicine, communications and physical education — there is a paucity of information about wrong breathing habits. The asthmatic does not need breathing exercises — he needs breathing *education*."

Temporomandibular Joint (TMJ) Disorders

Dental restorative techniques, such as reconstruction and bonding, have advanced tremendously over the years. To ensure that this costly and time-consuming dental work won't be undone by the patient's habitual mis-use patterns, such as grinding or gnashing of teeth while sleeping, a growing number of dentists refer these patients to Alexander teachers. Dr. Stanley Knebelman, a prominent Philadelphia dental surgeon, reports on his experience:

> "In my work with patients suffering TMJ disorders, I find there is *always* an accompanying misuse of the head and neck muscles as well as the muscles associated with oral functioning. It is not enough simply to restore or correct dental deformities. This does nothing to change the harmful misuse patterns that lie at the root of the problem. The only really effective treatment for TMJ patients requires a cooperative effort between the TMJ therapist — the dentist — and a skilled specialist in movement reeducation — a teacher of the Alexander Technique."

Migraine

Migraine headaches rarely occur in isolation. They are almost always accompanied by excessive tension in the muscles of the scalp, face, eyes, neck and throat. This is the area where tension often first builds up before spreading out to the rest of the body, and it is one of the first areas to release during Alexander lessons. The Technique therefore can sometimes have an almost immediate effect on migraines. Like other teachers, I've taught a number of pupils whose migraines disappeared after two or three sessions. In large measure, this relief from pain was due to their increased sensitivity. They learned to detect, and so prevent, harmful tension in the head and neck area *before* it could grow into the painful symptoms of a full blown migraine attack.

Most other methods of alleviating migraines focus on releasing tense muscles individually. This may well provide some temporary relief, but usually fails to deal with the use of these muscles as part of a habit set affecting the body as a whole. As long as this underlying pattern is allowed to continue, the migraine sufferer will still be easily susceptible to future attacks.

Overall Fitness

Many eminent medical investigators, among them Dr. Wilfred Barlow, referred to earlier, have found that mis-use of the body plays a major role in causing and perpetuating arthritis, rheumatism, gastro-intestinal conditions and even some sexual dysfunctions.

This isn't really surprising when you think about it. Mis-use generates abnormal pressures on joints and on the vertebrae of the spinal column, distorts body shape and hinders the operation of vital organs. And because it takes a lot of work to keep muscles overly contracted, locking whole areas of the body into a fixed position, the body is forced to expend its energy in harmful directions. One result can be a feeling of chronic fatigue; another is a weakening of the body's defenses against disease.

The human body is designed so that each internal organ operates at peak efficiency when it is allowed to easily fill its share of space. Because there is no empty, wasted space, any distortion in the body's shape forces internal organs up against one another, making it difficult for them to perform their specialized functions. Just as serious, the pressures produced by this unnatural squeezing hinder the crucially important circulatory flows connecting the organs with each other and the rest of the body.

Helping pupils to improve their overall functioning can therefore produce a dramatic improvement in health. What might be called the "Alexander approach" to health and well-being has been nicely expressed by Eric de Peyer, an English teacher of the Technique for over half a century:

> "The Alexander Technique approaches the problem of physical and mental health in an indirect way. No attempt is made to *treat* any particular symptom (in any case few teachers of the method are likely to be qualified to do this) but rather to establish the positive conditions for health. This is analogous to tidying up an untidy room in order to find a missing object rather than searching for it directly and probably rending the room untidier still in the process. The indirect way may take a little longer, but it is more certain, will render further losses less likely, and will have accomplished something useful even if the missing object remains unfound. Also it may happen that something lost long since and which had been forgotten may turn up. It has, too, the further important advantage that one will at last become fully aware of the contents of the room in a way that one had not been before."

We know from experience that even a short vacation or a change of scene can be therapeutic. What the Alexander Technique offers us is the possibility of a lifetime vacation from the harmful effects of mis-use.

Emotions and the Alexander Technique

Our entire language is permeated with phrases attesting to the link between the state of our body and our emotions: "stiff-necked", "level-headed", "pulled down", "depressed", "carrying the weight of the world on her shoulders", "he has no backbone", and so on. And most of us can get a pretty good idea of a friend's emotional state by observing him. Hunched shoulders and a drooped posture tell one story, a light bouncy walk quite another.

Of course physical tension can, on occasion, be a kind of natural anesthetic which we use to protect ourselves in situations where we feel vulnerable. This is what psychiatrist Wilheim Reich referred to as "armoring", an apt description of both the process and its result.

One of the great strengths of the Alexander Technique is that changes are never forced. Pupils improve at a pace that is guided by their own "body wisdom". In this way, the Technique avoids the potential harm of sudden or violent releases of blocked emotions that can result from too quick a stripping away of psychological "armor" which, after all, is there for a purpose and can only usefully be surrendered when it is no longer needed.

Many years ago, in commenting about the effects of the Technique, Aldous Huxely made the following observation:

> "If you teach an individual first to be aware
> of his physical organism and then to use it as it
> was meant to be used you can often change his
> entire attitude to life and cure his neurotic
> tendencies."

At the time, this idea was probably considered a bit far-fetched by some. Today, of course, medical science increasingly recognizes the powerful link between emotional and physical well-being, and it no longer seems surprising that for many pupils, the mental and emotional benefits of their lessons are at least as important for them as the more obvious physical changes they experience. Indeed, because the improvements in their physical condition are due largely to their own efforts, pupils frequently experience a feeling of greater self confidence, a sense of at last being able to really take charge of themselves and cope effectively with the inevitable stresses of life.

Performers and the Alexander Technique

Ever since Alexander first began teaching, performers have gravitated to the Alexander Technique. Among the many who have publicly endorsed the Technique in recent years are Paul Newman, Julie Andrews, Nina Foch, John Cleese, Anthony Perkins, Joanne Woodward and Joel Grey.

A growing number of schools and universities are now offering courses in the Alexander Technique as part of performance training. A partial list includes:

Guildhall School of Music, London
The Julliard School
The Royal Academy of Dramatic Art, London
Los Angeles Philharmonic Orchestral Training Program
The Royal College of Music, London
University of California
Stratford Festival, Ontario
The London Academy of Music and Dramatic Art
Boston University
Brussels Royal Conservatory Theatre
American Dance Festival

This interest in the Technique on the part of performers and their teachers reflects their clear understanding of the link between the way they use their body and the quality of their performance.

Obviously a singer who tenses her neck and shoulder muscles will not be able to produce the best sound possible. Nor will a violinist whose fingers, shoulders and wrists are stiff. Conversely, dancers who use their bodies well and move with natural grace and ease look more appealing and are less likely to suffer injuries. Likewise, an actor attempting to convince the audience that he *is* the character portrayed will want to use his body in a way which appears entirely convincing, without doing harm to himself. A striking example of the opposite was sadly provided by Charles Laughton who, in his brilliant film portrayal of "The Hunchback of Notre Dame", did himself permanent physical injury.

Performers also have special needs for the Alexander Technique because of the unusual demands they place on themselves. Singers, musicians, dancers, athletes and actors all spend long hours rehearsing or practicing, repeating the same movements over and over. Then too there is the stress of appearing before an audience or camera. Furthermore, the intense competition for jobs in these fields can easily add to a performer's anxieties.

The Performer in All of Us

Of course, entertainers and athletes aren't the only ones who must rely on performance skills to carry out their work successfully. Personal impressions play a major role in a wide variety of jobs — sales, public relations, hospitality and medicine, to name but a few — and many people who work in these fields have derived invaluable professional benefits from lessons in the Alexander Technique. We all know that the individual who habitually slouches, or who appears tense and ill at ease, makes a far less favorable impression on a potential client, or on his boss, than one who has an easy, upright and confident manner.

In most occupations, in fact, the ability to mobilize all our physical, mental and emotional resources is at least as important as our mastery of the specific job skills required. My previous profession, economic research and analysis, was one that required very little contact with the public. Yet even here, the people who rose to the top were frequently *not* those with the greatest technical skills. They typically combined a basic, often quite ordinary, analytical capability with a special talent to easily sense and respond to the needs and desires of others in the organization.

As might be expected, the Technique has proven itself to be particularly helpful for those working in fields which require special communications skills. Some time ago, a successful trial lawyer came to me for lessons. She originally complained of migraines and sleeplessness. The relief of these symptoms was accompanied by an unexpected dividend: a dramatic improvement in her performance in court.

Her job requires much more than legal expertise and thorough preparation. She is required to relate effectively to the judge, other lawyers, the jury, witnesses, and courtroom officials, often at the same time. She must also send and receive verbal and non-verbal "body language" messages efficiently, respond quickly, convey sincerity, and of course always present her client's case in the most favorable light.

What surprised her the most was that as she became better at winning cases, she also found her courtroom work easier, less stressful and a lot more enjoyable.

For many years, I have been fascinated by the special skills demonstrated by sign language interpreters. Recently,

I had a chance to interview Catherine Kettrick, who works in an interpreter training program and is herself a qualified Alexander teacher in Seattle. She reports that the Technique helps her own interpreting in two distinct ways:

"First, it helps me to think more clearly and understand more quickly what a person is saying. Because I am not wasting energy with unnecessary tension, I literally have more time to understand a message and reconstruct it in the other language. Second, if I am sign interpreting, my movements are much easier and clearer so the person watching me can understand me easily, and I do not become tired so quickly."

Fit For Life

A growing number of people are coming to the Alexander Technique not because of a specific problem, but to improve their general health and well being. Sometimes they are seeking a way to *avoid* problems — they don't, for instance, want to wait until they suffer backache before improving their posture.

Others have come for lessons in order to develop their *competence*, a word which has been nicely defined as "the free exercise of dexterity and intelligence in the completion of tasks." Following the classical ideal "Know thyself". they want to understand how they function — and how they can *improve* their functioning. They have become intrigued and excited by the journey of self-discovery and self-development that the Alexander Technique can provide.

By now, you probably have some idea of how the Technique could be of help to you. In Chapter Five, you'll learn how to locate a qualified teacher. But first, in the next chapter, let's take a look at what actually goes on during an Alexander lesson.

Dave is in his forties, is blind, and lives in Columbus, Ohio, where he has a successful career as a piano tuner.

"Piano tuning is a job where you often have to use a certain amount of force. And you have to repeat the same kind of action over and over again. You're always using your right hand to pull on a tool which turns a little pin. You need extreme accuracy to get it just right. With the effort I was making — both mental and physical — to be really precise, I knew I was tensing myself up to make this one tiny movement. Also you sometimes have to work around the physical mass of the piano which can get you into some very awkward positions.

"Anyway, I started getting a lot of discomfort in my neck and shoulders, and my arms as well, especially while I was working. That's how I heard about the Technique — I mentioned the pain to one of my clients, a professional pianist, while I was working for him. Like a lot of musicians, he's had courses of Alexander lessons to get rid of tension and improve his performance. He thought the Technique could probably help me, too. I was getting so worried about the pain and the effect it could have on my work that I decided it was worth a try.

"I went for a private lesson with a teacher he recommended. I didn't have much idea what to expect, but I certainly have a striking memory of that first lesson.

"With none of the visual information that sighted people get all the time, I guess somebody blind like myself tends to be more sensitive to touch. And we're certainly used to being touched — you'd probably be amazed at how many times in the course of an average week some well meaning stranger grabs hold of me without saying a word and tries to walk me through a door, across a street, on

and off the bus — whether I want to or not!

"*But the way that teacher used his hands was unique in my experience. It was a very light touch, say on the neck or upper back, but I felt this amazing release. With his hand on the back of my neck, I felt as if I were growing a foot taller, as if he had lifted me off the ground. No force or manipulation in it, though — this was definitely* not *being grabbed hold of or shoved around.*

"*He got me to walk around the room, all the time bringing my attention, both with words and touch, to what I was doing to myself as I moved. That was a revelation. I suddenly realized how unconscious I was of my own movement patterns and habits. We started table work in the second lesson and again I had this whole new sensation of lightness and ease.*

"*I very soon realized that the most important thing at first was to use the Technique to re-educate myself concerning my general way of functioning, rather than concentrating right away on my problems at work. It's a little like learning a new language and realizing you need to understand some basics before you can apply it to a specific situation — unless you're just going to memorize a few phrases, with no real idea of what you're saying.*

"*So, for two or three months we worked on general things like walking, sitting, standing, speaking, and it was towards the end of that period that we worked specifically on my piano tuning and how I used myself during that. By then I was sufficiently familiar with this new Alexander body 'language' really to understand what he was telling me and showing me with his hands. My work certainly got easier and more enjoyable — and naturally less tiring. An important part of this was that I felt an ease in breathing, a kind of opening up in my chest, that was completely new to me.*

"*I have to say that, apart from the purely practical aspects, I discovered that one of the basic things I had to learn for the first time in my life was how to be easier on myself. I don't know whether it's because I'm blind, or just the kind of person I am, or both, but I'd always felt that the only way to achieve anything was to struggle really hard and push myself. Of course, there is a place for that kind of effort in life, but the Alexander Technique has demonstrated to me that there's also a way of growing and learning by being patient and gentle and just letting go. I think the profoundest changes happened when I realized that."*

4

THE ALEXANDER LESSON

When I speak to new pupils on the telephone before their first lesson, I find they often have questions about what will go on during the lesson and, more generally, about the teaching process itself. In this chapter, I'll answer the ones that come up most often. But first, I would like to allay some common — and quite unfounded — anxieties, under the general heading of:

What Not to Expect

For a start, you don't remove your clothes. In fact, in the winter chill of his London office, Alexander himself often taught people who were still wearing their heavy outdoor coats. (Fortunately, with the modern advances in central heating — compared to what was available in England fifty years ago — we don't usually have to go to that extreme now!)

Nor is any kind of special clothing required — though as table work often forms part of the lesson, women pupils usually feel more comfortable wearing slacks, or jeans, rather than a skirt.

As you've probably been gathering from reading the personal accounts, Alexander lessons are not painful. There is nothing physically aggressive about the work. On the contrary, it is a process of allowing the pupil to release tension — *and* the harmful habits that were responsible for it — at the pace that suits him, individually.

This brings me to another extremely important point: Alexander lessons, whether individual private ones or group work, are in no way competitive. Your teacher *will* observe your patterns of movement in order to find out as much about them as possible, but there is nothing "judgmental" in this. His aim is always to put you as much at ease as possible, which of course considerably helps the learning process. A teacher will never feed your anxieties — and consequently your tension — by making you feel that you're somehow "getting it wrong".

Actually, you'll be even less inclined to feel self conscious if you bear in mind that the teacher has been through the same process himself. Some of today's finest Alexander teachers were themselves drawn to the Technique because of quite serious physical problems of their own, caused by injuries, childhood diseases and the like. In any case, you can be certain that your teacher is not someone with a mysterious innate talent for good use. His own use has been improved — and probably still is being improved — by years of training during which, just like you, he has had to overcome harmful habits of posture and movement. He *knows* how normal those habits feel, how unfamiliar it feels at first to let them go and how easy it is to slide back into them. So there is no question of him having the impatience or incomprehension of the "natural genius" who cannot appreciate the plodding efforts of the less talented!

In keeping with this attitude, he will probably encourage you to ask questions, whenever you wish. When any kind of process is very new to us, we're often afraid of asking "silly" questions. But with the Alexander Technique — as in many other fields — the "simplest" questions from the "beginner" can often turn out to be among the most profound.

Now for those telephone questions.

Where Do Lessons Take Place?

Many teachers work in their own homes. A home environment not only helps you to feel comfortable but also underscores the fact that the Alexander Technique is not something to be isolated from normal daily life and activities.

Other teachers prefer to work in an office or studio and, of course, teachers employed by theatre companies, music schools and the like, to work with their faculty and students, usually teach on the premises.

Will the Teacher Diagnose my Problem?

There is no medical diagnosis in any Alexander Technique lesson. On the contrary, your teacher will ask you to check with your own doctor about anything that might indicate a medical problem.

However, as you might expect, your teacher will ask you why you've come for lessons. He will probably inquire about your work and your leisure time activities in order to build up as complete a picture as possible of what is contributing to your present patterns of use.

What Does the Teacher Do?

As I've already said, during the lesson your teacher will

be observing your posture and movement patterns. He will also supplement this visual information in a very important way by using his hands, gently placing them on your neck, shoulders, back and so on. There is nothing embarrassing about this as care is taken never to make contact with overtly sexual areas of the body. The teacher is using his hands in order to get more refined information about your patterns of breathing and moving.

To help him with this, he will probably ask you to perform some simple movements — perhaps walking, or standing up or sitting down in a chair — while his hands are kept in easy contact with your body. He does this to find out as much as he can about your patterns of use.

As you work together, he may further supplement this information by asking you questions about *your* perception of what is happening — what you can sense or what you are thinking about. Obviously, the more information he has, the better he is able to help you.

Another reason for questioning you in this way is to encourage you to become aware of the connection between your thoughts and your movements. After all, your brain ultimately controls the actions of your muscles and your teacher wants you to learn as much as possible about how your complete mind/body mechanism operates.

At the same time that the teacher's hands are *gathering* information, they will also be *conveying* information to you. The teacher's hands will gently "speak" to muscles in your body that are overly tense and encourage them to begin to release. This is a very subtle process and one you may not consciously notice at first.

Naturally, teachers vary somewhat in their approaches to teaching. Just like any other group of professionals, there are variations due to differences in personality and style of training. Some teachers may talk and explain more at first; others prefer to spend most of the time during the first lessons simply helping you to get a new experience of ease and flexibility. Similarly, some teachers emphasize a few, fairly basic movements — allowing the effect to carry over into all your activities — while others prefer to work with you in a wide variety of applications.

These differences are not in themselves particularly important. What really matters are the practical benefits you derive from the lessons, and take into your daily life.

What is "Tablework"?

At some point during the lesson, your teacher may ask you to lie on your back on a table, with some support under your head and with your knees bent. This is the "Alexander lying-down position", sometimes also referred to as "semi-supine". In this position, the effects of gravity are minimized, enabling your teacher to help you achieve greater release than might otherwise be possible. Your teacher will again use his hands to help you free over-stiffened muscles in the legs, arms, torso — and particularly in the neck, which is where tension often originates before spreading out to other areas of the body.

What Will I Feel During a Lesson?

Perhaps nothing at all to begin with — and that is no cause for concern. The process of release and change can be a very subtle one and people have different degrees of sensitivity. It is possible for important changes to be underway without your being at first aware of them. However, it is also quite likely that you will notice some new sensations even during the first lesson. Pupils frequently make comments like: "I feel taller", "I feel lighter", "I'm breathing more fully", "My head seems to be floating", and so on.

From an early age, most of us have been physically tensing ourselves up in a whole variety of ways until we have practically forgotten what it is to move in a balanced, graceful manner. When we begin to let go of this tension, the resultant feelings of release are naturally unfamiliar at first.

In his book, *Body Awareness in Action*, Frank Pierce Jones gives a good description of what this can be like. He was having his first lesson in the Technique and his teacher was guiding him from a sitting to a standing position. This is what he wrote about it:

"The most striking aspect of the movement was the sensory effect of lightness that it induced. The feeling had not been present at the start, nor had it been suggested to me; it was clearly a direct result of the movement. While it lasted, everything I did, including breathing, became easier. After a short time the effect faded away, leaving me, however, with the certainty that I had glimpsed a new world of experience which had more to offer than the limited set of movement patterns, attitudes, and responses to which I was accustomed."

Most of us have indeed become accustomed to dealing with tension simply by shifting it around — changing our seating position, for example, to take some of the pressure off one area, only to find it building up somewhere else. In marked contrast to this, the Alexander Technique does not get us to *rearrange* long standing tension patterns; it teaches us to *release* them. Hence the dramatic differences we often perceive in ourselves, and the striking insights we gain into the physical stresses we have for years been unnecessarily inflicting upon ourselves.

How Soon Will I Notice Changes?

Pupils almost always notice changes within the first
two or three weeks of lessons. What makes it possible for
changes to occur as quickly and smoothly as they do is
that the Technique is really a process of *re*-learning, or
re-acquiring, the poise, flexibility and easy coordination
we once had as children, but which, over time, have fallen
prey to the stresses of life.

To some extent, these early changes seem to occur
with very little effort on the part of the pupil, but as he
continues with the Technique he learns to make a more
conscious effort on his own behalf. He becomes more
aware of harmful habits, better able to sense their onset
and turn them aside, well before they build up to their full
force and take control of him.

This is why Alexander teachers are so firm about using
the words "teacher" and "pupil", or "student". We view
the Technique, as Alexander did, not as a treatment applied to a passive patient, but as a process of education
aimed at enabling the pupil to take responsibility for himself and, eventually, to play the major role in his own
progress. The aim is always to equip the student with a
lasting skill derived from an increased sensitivity to, and
knowledge about, his own body and the way his thinking
directs his movements. The aim is most definitely *not* to
make him dependent on us to "fix him up".

Lessons are always a co-operative project. The learning
has to be done by the pupil, although the teacher provides
a lot of help, especially at the start when the pupil is ex-
ploring ways of thinking and moving which are quite unfamiliar to him. As time goes by, the pupil increasingly
becomes his own teacher and eventually no longer has
need of any teacher other than himself. As Marjorie
Barstow, a senior American teacher of the Technique aptly
puts it: "The teacher draws the map, but the pupil explores

the territory."

This captures the process very well: without a "map", it would be all too easy to get lost in what could easily become a hopelessly time-consuming and frustrating search — remember Alexander's *ten years* of trial and error! On the other hand, a "map" is certainly no substitute for the actual exploration itself.

How Long Are Lessons — And How Many Will I Need?

A lesson usually lasts between thirty and forty-five minutes. This is in keeping with the findings of education researchers, who consider it to be about the maximum time span over which people can effectively absorb new information. One would certainly expect this to be true for an Alexander lesson, where the new information is both verbal and kinesthetic. In fact, a skilled teacher can convey a great deal of information in that time.

The Alexander Technique is a powerful tool with a wide range of applications. In many ways, however, the process of actually learning it is comparable to the acquisition of any new skill. It's not surprising, therefore, that the number of lessons needed varies quite a bit from person to person and there is nothing standardized about the teaching process, no "Level A" or "Level B" or anything like that.

It will probably take several lessons for both you and your teacher to get an idea of how quickly you will progress, although the teacher can often tell a good deal in the first lesson. Another, even more important reason that the number of lessons cannot be specified is that it depends — as with other skills — on how far you want to take it. That can't be predicted at the start of the process, not even by the pupil. Attempting to gauge the number of lessons in advance is a little like wanting to know how many lessons are needed, let's say, to learn French. The answer would depend of course on your linguistic ability, but even more on the *level* of proficiency you wanted to reach.

However, having said this, I can at least give you a rough idea of what I have found to be a fairly typical pattern for my own pupils — and those of other teachers as well. We find — with many exceptions, of course, in both directions — that the majority of pupils come to us for a few months, taking between twenty and forty lessons in that period and then, perhaps, come back for "refresher" lessons, or groups of lessons, from time to time.

At the start, pupils are usually urged to come for lessons fairly frequently, perhaps two or three times a week if that's at all possible. This is because the new approach to movement, and to thinking about movement, which they are learning, is a bit unfamiliar at first and may need a little extra help to become established. Later on in the process, pupils often find they can continue to progress quite well with lessons spaced a week or more apart.

What About Group Work?

Like psychotherapy, the Alexander Technique originated with one-to-one work and most teachers today continue to teach in this way. But just as we now know that individual therapy can take place in a group setting, so too, some Alexander teachers have found that by working with individuals in a group setting, they can help far more people than would ever have been possible with individual lessons. Indeed, this is the basis on which many Alexander teacher training courses are organized.

Experience has shown that under the right circumstances, group work can be a very effective way of teaching. The teacher, of course, has to be good at establishing rapport with the group and not everyone who is a good teacher at the indivdual level will automatically be good at teaching groups — or necessarily wish to do so.

The success of group work also depends on the personality of the pupils. They have to be able to feel at home in a group setting in order to derive benefit from it. Each pupil also has to be willing to take a lot of responsibility for learning, right from the start. Sometimes, group work is most effective *after* the pupil has had at least a few private lessons, but this certainly is not always the case.

One notable advantage of group work, which teachers skilled in this way of working utilize, is that pupils learn from observing the others in the group. It is of course part of the teacher's job to ensure that this process of mutual observation remains non-competitive and non-judgmental.

It goes without saying that group work may not be the best approach for pupils who have very serious problems and who therefore have a special need of the teacher's undivided attention.

Are There Special Exercises?

The Alexander Technique is a method of enhancing our ability to carry out any activity, whether it be simply standing or sitting, doing routine day-to-day tasks, or engaging in demanding athletic or performance events. A student of the Technique doesn't get better and better at "doing Alexander" as an end in itself. What he does gain over time is the ability to apply more effectively, and to a wider range of activities, the knowledge he has gained during lessons.

So, with one or two very minor exceptions which we need not consider here, there is no such thing as an "Alexander exercise". Indeed, the phrase is really a contradiction in terms. Exercises usually involve repeating the same movements over and over again and, as we have seen, by

themselves they contribute nothing to changing underlying habit patterns. The Alexander Technique can help
you to *improve* the way you do things — precisely so that
you won't have to do them over and over in the same way.

Of course, some pupils may want to continue an exercise program already begun, or perhaps start a new one.
The Alexander Technique can help them to exercise in an
efficient, coordinated — and *pleasurable* — way, with minimum risk of injury or harmful wear and tear on their
bodies.

Many Alexander teachers, myself included, recom-
mend to their pupils that they spend some time each day
in the Alexander lying down position, described earlier.
This is not really an exercise, but it does encourage a
lengthening and release of over-tightened muscles throughout your body, particularly those of the neck and torso,
and can be an extremely effective means of augmenting
the lessons themselves.

In general, tension is released more easily when you no
longer have to maintain your upright posture. Many people
are surprised to learn they are taller in the morning than at
night. (You can easily verify this by having someone measure your height before going to bed, and then first thing
the next morning.) The difference is due to the overnight
release of tension that had built up during the day, con-
tracting your body in on itself.

The Alexander lying down position encourages this
process of lengthening and release even more effectively.
Alexander first used this position in the early part of the
century as a supplement to his teaching. In recent years,
doctors, chiropractors and physiotherapists have begun to
suggest it for people suffering back pain, although they
sometimes neglect to include support under the head,
without which much of the benefit is lost.

One pupil of mine, an advertising executive who works
all day in a particularly stressful environment, finds that

the half hour between arriving home from work and having dinner with his family is an ideal time to do his lying down. It quickly replaced his previous method of unwinding — drinking a large scotch and soda — and both he and his family are very pleased with the change.

Will I Have To Do Any Homework?

People with a busy schedule, who are considering taking Alexander lessons, are sometimes worried they'll have to spend many hours a day "practicing their Alexander". Actually, apart from the lessons themselves, the only other activity which takes up any additional time is the few minutes a day spent in the Alexander lying down position. Students often find they need less sleep at night, or are able to dispense with customary naps, so in all probability there will be no real loss of time.

The most important activity outside lessons is the application of what you learn to your daily activities, whatever they may be. This is a gradual process and it certainly does not require you to spend the whole day thinking about your use — *that* would soon become a tedious chore! But as you become more sensitive to your body, you will become better able to prevent unwanted habit patterns from asserting themselves. You will find your attention gently drawn to potential troublespots and restrictions and you'll then be able to more easily re-direct your energies to encourage the free flow of your body's movements.

At times, you may find yourself engaging in some deliberate experimentation. This is exactly what Alexander did during his early investigations. Today, of course, the process of learning is far quicker because, unlike Alexander, you'll have the assistance of a teacher who has been through the same process himself. He can help you avoid mistakes and, during each lesson, take you further along the path of self-discovery than you could probably go on your own.

Sometimes, Alexander "homework" can have immediate benefits. A pupil of one of my colleagues, who had only had a half dozen lessons or so, was involved in a serious automobile accident. She was waiting at an intersection for the light to change when, in her rear view mirror, she saw a car suddenly coming at her from behind. She couldn't drive forward because of the traffic and there was certainly no way to get out of her car before the inevitable collision. She noticed that the muscles of her neck were tensing and she had the presence of mind to release them, as she had been learning to do in her lessons. Although there was a fair amount of property damage, both she and her doctor were amazed that she had suffered no whiplash or other injury.

Alexander's method of teaching has proved its usefulness in a great variety of ways. We are therefore extremely fortunate that he developed a way to pass his understanding and skills on to others so that today there are qualified teachers in many parts of the world. The next chapter will tell you how you can locate a teacher and begin to learn the Alexander Technique yourself.

Margaret is a housewife in her sixties, who lives in Baltimore.

"It was my daughter who first got me to take Alexander lessons. She's a singer and I knew she took lessons in the Alexander Technique to help her professionally. I was real surprised when she said it would be good for me to take some, because I thought it was just for musicians.

"I had various problems — physical ones, I mean — but I'd had them as long as I could remember and they just seemed part of the way I was. I'd had asthma since I was a

child. I just thought I was stuck with it. And I always knew that I slouched — pretty badly — but it just seemed the natural thing for me. Mind you, I hated catching sight of myself in those full-length mirrors they have in stores. I always looked even more hunched and hollow chested than I thought. You know how that makes you look real old — and sort of defeated? Seeing myself like that always made me straighten up, but that was so darn uncomfortable that it would only last for a minute or two and back down I'd go again!

"Then there was my breathing. Even apart from the asthma, it had always been real shallow and anything that needed a little more energy, like walking up the stairs, really took it out of me. But again, I just thought, 'That's the way I am'.

"I enjoy sewing — I'm pretty good with a needle and thread and I even teach quilting at the local community college. One evening when I was sitting at home sewing, my daughter said: 'Mom, you just don't have to hunch over it like that — you're using so much energy pulling yourself down!'

"She really made me stop and notice for the first time how tensed up I was — and sewing was something I did for pleasure and relaxation! She even teased me a little. 'Look,' she said, 'how much does that thin little needle weigh? But your're gripping it like it was a pneumatic drill!'

"Anyway, she eventually got me to give the Alexander Technique a try — and I certainly haven't regretted it. Almost immediately — I mean after two or three weeks — I noticed this big change in my breathing. It was deeper, yet so much easier, and this seemed to lead naturally to a real sharp decline in my asthma attacks. There was also a change in my posture — although I guess that wasn't really a separate thing — the breathing, the asthma, the slouching were all really part of the same problem. This new posture wasn't the old 'straightening up' kind of thing I used to

do — for about a minute at a time! — but a real natural-feeling upward movement.

"I noticed that my chest was a lot less caved in. It felt as though it had opened up for the first time in years. My teacher told me that's why my breathing was so much easier — I wasn't clenching my rib cage so much anymore. I still get the occasional asthma attack, but when I feel it coming on, I can generally stop it by releasing the tension the way I learned in my Alexander lessons.

"All in all, the most important change is that I now understand what I have been doing all my life. I'd always thought of slouching as 'not making an effort' — something I felt sort of guilty about, but the effort needed to straighten up usually seemed too hard to make. Now I can see how much work goes into slouching and I realize that good posture — and all the wonderful things that go with it — is really just letting go of all that unnecessary tension. I think I'd gotten so used to all that tension before that it just felt normal to me.

"The Alexander Technique has certainly made me feel years younger. No, my wrinkles didn't just go away overnight! But this much I can say for sure — at my age, to move around and do things with this much grace and ease is a whole lot more rejuvenating than one of those face lifts or a bunch of fancy new clothes!"

5

GETTING STARTED

A few years after I began teaching, a local newspaper ran a story about ways to alleviate back pain. It included a reference to the Alexander Technique and gave my phone number. Among the calls I received was one from a retired police officer who, many years earlier, had read one of Alexander's books. He had been spending long hours sitting in a patrol car and had developed severe pain in his lower back which failed to respond to any of the treatments he had tried. Alexander's method seemed to him a sensible approach, but he had no idea where to find a teacher. He saw the article quite by chance and so, at last, he was able to learn how to put into practice the ideas he had read about so long ago. Ironically, it turned out that he lived almost directly across the street from me!

As a result of several experiences like that one, and of problems which have sometimes been caused by untrained individuals claiming to teach the Alexander Technique, I decided that the subject of how to locate a qualified teacher was important enough to warrant a whole chapter in this book. But first, I'd like to say a word or two about the training process an Alexander teacher has gone through, and what distinguishes it from the training requirements

for other treatments, disciplines, therapies etc., that you
may have heard about.

Training the Alexander Teacher

I referred earlier to the very high standards that F. M.
Alexander insisted upon when training other teachers.
These standards are still upheld today and rigorously en-
forced by our three major professional societies:. the
British-based Society of Teachers for the Alexander Tech-
nique (STAT), the North American Society of Teachers of
the Alexander Technique (NASTAT), and the American
Guild of Teachers of the Alexander Technique (AGTAT).

To be recognized by STAT, NASTAT or AGTAT,
Alexander teacher training courses must satisfy their strin-
gent requirements: three years of full time training; a
teacher-student ratio of at least one to five; one course
director with a minimum of seven years' teaching experience; at least one other with a minimum of five years'
experience.

The training process itself is very much like an ap-
prenticeship. (In fact, a few teachers fulfill their training
requirements by studying individually, for several years,
with a master teacher of the Technique.) Class sizes are
quite small — usually no more than fifteen or twenty students, at the very most — so that everyone has ample opportunity for personal instruction. Often, towards the end
of the course, trainees will do some practice teaching
under the watchful eyes (and guiding hands) of an experienced faculty member.

Much of a trainee's time, particularly in the first two
years, is devoted to refining their own manner of use. To
be able to teach the Technique, they must have undergone
sufficient re-education themselves to be able to accurately
sense malfunctioning in a pupil, and to provide the kines-

thetic and verbal information necessary to help him bring about an improvement.

Indeed, it is the improved use of themselves that ultimately makes it possible for Alexander teachers to help others so effectively. "Those who can, do, and those who cannot, teach" may be true in some other fields; it most definitely is *not* the case with the Alexander Technique.

Teaching the Individual

As you can see, there is a world of difference between the training of an Alexander teacher and that of so many "body therapists" of one kind or another who are launched "qualified" on the public after a few months — or even a few weekends — of "training", often in large classes with little or no personal instruction. Moreover, Alexander teachers usually regard their three years training as merely a foundation on which to build. Throughout their careers, many of them attend special courses with master teachers in order to further refine their teaching skills.

There is no avoiding the fact that it takes time and dedication to develop the necessary sensitivity and adroitness to be an effective teacher of the Alexander Technique. The protracted, in-depth training of such a teacher reflects the fact that human movement and posture patterns are far too complex to be well understood in a short time.

For instance, every individual has a "range of flexibility" within which he can make constructive improvements in his movement patterns. Trying to push too rapidly beyond that range is always counterproductive, and generally results in, at best, a stiff parody of what the Technique aims for. Of course, a pupil's range of flexibility itself expands with lessons, often quite dramatically. So the task of an Alexander teacher is to help you as much as possible within the limits of your present abilities, *and* to assist you in widening those limits in a way, and at a speed, that is consistent with your overall well-being.

Many of the newer therapies which have proliferated in recent years miss subtleties of this kind completely. Often their goal is to have you conform to some sort of "ideal" pattern which bears no relationship to you as a unique individual.

To take just one example, there is much talk these days about proper "body alignment". And it is certainly true that most pupils of the Alexander Technique find that their posture improves with lessons, becoming increasingly symmetrical and balanced. This is one of the more obvious, visible results of their generally improved use of themselves. However, any direct attempt to mold your body into "perfect" alignment — as though there were such a thing — would do you no good whatsoever, and might even be harmful, if the myriad of interrelationships within your body, and between your mind and body, are not taken into account at the same time.

We all know from observation and experience that we human beings are an extraordinarily diverse lot, differing widely in physiology and temperament. It is not surprising, therefore, that constructive and genuinely helpful changes in ourselves, of any kind, can *never* be accomplished merely by following a "formula", or a simplistic set of rules or exercises.

Beware of Impostors

With the growing interest in the Technique, the number of qualified teachers has increased dramatically in the past few years. When I began taking lessons in the mid 1970's, there were only three teachers in all of Canada. Now there are nearly three dozen. I was lucky in that my teacher lived in the same city as I did, but many of his pupils traveled a hundred miles or more each way; some came to town for a week or two at a time, just to have a series of lessons.

The increase in teachers has been worldwide, from a few hundred a decade ago to well over a thousand today. During the next five years, the number of teachers is expected to reach more than twice that number. With this rapid expansion, and the growing public awareness of the Technique, the inevitable has happened: a number of untrained and unscrupulous individuals cashing in on its excellent reputation and presenting themselves to the public as teachers of the Technique.

This is a problem our profession shares with many others — psychotherapy, marriage counseling, consulting and some other teaching fields, for example. Because the Alexander Technique is an educational process, not a medical intervention, there is no *legal* recourse against these unqualified opportunists.

A somewhat different problem sometimes comes up when teachers of subjects like dance, acting or singing, who themselves have benefited from Alexander lessons, try to teach the Technique to their own pupils. Their intentions are often good, but because Alexander teaching *looks* deceptively simple, they fail to appreciate just how much training and practice it takes to do it effectively.

Clearly, it *is* very helpful for people in these fields to have some personal experience with the Technique. It helps the teaching of their own discipline, and can make it possible for them to spot problems in their students' coordination and balance that are restricting their progress and that a qualified Alexander Technique teacher could help with. Indeed, that is how most performance teachers make use of the Technique. However, there are a few who actually purport to teach it, and that is quite a different matter.

Finding a Qualified Teacher

Fortunately today there is a simple way to locate a
fully qualified teacher. STAT, NASTAT and AGTAT will
supply a complete listing of all their affiliated teachers.
The societies' addresses and phone numbers are located at
the back of this book. So too are those of a number of national societies which are affiliated with STAT. In addition
to providing teachers' lists, professional societies are often
the best source of up-to-date information about activities
of interest to Alexander students — talks, demonstrations,
residential courses and the like.

If No Teacher is Nearby

Should you find that there is no teacher available in
your area, there are three things you can do:
First, attend a residential course. These are now of-
fered in many countries. They run for a week or two at a
time and it is possible to learn quite a lot in that period because the teaching is concentrated and there are usually
several Alexander teachers working as a team with the
group. The courses are usually held in pleasant locations
and are an enjoyable and beneficial way to get started in
the Technique, or to refresh one's knowledge Indeed,
some teachers believe this is one of the best ways to learn
about the Technique. Information on how you can find
the dates and locations of these courses is provided at the
back of this book, immediately following the list of professional societies.
Second, travel to a teacher. It is not uncommon for
pupils to spend a week or two in a city or town which has
an Alexander teacher, taking a daily series of lessons during that period. This is often done in connection with business or vacation travel. Obviously it is important to arrange

the lessons well in advance of your trip.

Finally, bring a teacher to you. Nowadays, some Alexander teachers regularly spend time away from their home base. It will require a certain amount of organizing on your part, but if you can get a dozen or so people together and arrange accommodation and scheduling, it can be an excellent way to introduce the Technique into your community. As with residential courses, this solution offers the kind of concentrated instruction which works best for many pupils. Additionally, it is quite likely that someone in your area will, after having lessons in the Technique, decide to enroll in a training course. Then, in three years' time, you'll have your own local teacher.

What to Expect From Your Teacher

Teachers come from many different backgrounds. Most of them have had other careers before becoming Alexander teachers and, as you would expect, there is a wide variety of personalities represented in the profession.

As your teacher is someone who will be working very closely with you, it is important that you feel at ease with him. The teacher should, during a lesson, be there *for you*. That does not mean he or she does all the work. As we saw in the previous chapter, lessons are a cooperative venture and ultimately the learning has to be done by you. But you should certainly have a sense that your teacher is fully present to help you to learn as much and as quickly as you are capable of.

Above all, the teacher should be effective in helping you to discard your old, harmful habits. It is reassuring to know that with lessons in the Alexander Technique you'll soon become aware of the constructive changes you are making. You don't have to carry on with lessons for many weeks or months, taking it on trust that you are progressing. Within a short time, you will be aware of positive results — though sometimes those very first changes are noticed by your friends and relatives before you can sense them yourself.

Bear in mind, though, that the changes may not take place in the order that you expect, or that you might choose. For instance, an aching shoulder — someone's initial reason for coming for lessons — may have to wait for relief until other more fundamental changes take place, perhaps the freeing of the jaw, or neck, whose stiffness had gone unnoticed. As you can see from the personal accounts, pupils are frequently surprised by the unexpected ways in which the Technique works.

Pupils sometimes ask if there is an advantage in taking lessons with more than one teacher. From my own experience as a student and then a teacher, I would suggest staying with one person until you have established a good foundation in the principles and practice of the Technique. Teachers have their own individual way of working and a change could be confusing when you are still in the early stages of absorbing new ways of thinking and moving.

However, after you have become more familiar with the Technique, exposure to different teaching approaches can be extremely useful. Something which had been a bit puzzling can suddenly become clear when it is explained, or experienced, in a different way.

Do You Really Need a Teacher?

Prospective pupils sometimes inquire about the possibility of learning the Technique on their own. F. M. Alexander was, after all, his own teacher. In fact, with the dry humour characteristic of him, he was fond of remarking, "Anyone who does what I did, can do what I have done." And he meant exactly what he said.

But let's look at what that would mean in practical terms. Alexander spent *ten years* finding the solution to his own problem. Very little of that time was taken up with identifying the problem; it took him only a few months to observe that he was tightening his neck and stiffening his body whenever he began to speak. Most of that ten years was devoted to trying, over and over again, to devise a way to stop doing these things. According to his own account he made a lot of mistakes and went up a great many blind alleys. This is hardly surprising: he had no outside source of feedback — he had to depend entirely on himself.

> "Personally, I cannot speak with too much admiration — in the original sense of wonder as well as the sense of respect — of the persistence and thoroughness with which these extremely diligent observations and experiments were carried out."

That's what John Dewey had to say about the process Alexander went through in order to make his discoveries. It's a wonder to me that he was *ever* able to accomplish what he did by his own efforts alone. Teachers who knew him personally agree that he was a very special individual: talented and extraordinarily persevering. I doubt very much that many people, even if they had the time and motivation, could achieve by themselves what Alexander managed to do. Indeed, towards the end of his life, Alexander commented that in his experience, efforts to put his teaching into practice without expert help were seldom successful.

It must be said, however, that he did go as far as he possibly could in providing written guidance to those who were really serious about learning his Technique on their own. In a chapter entitled "Evolution of a Technique" in his third book, *The Use of The Self* (originally published in 1931), Alexander described in precise detail the process he went through to solve his voice problem. This chapter, along with his 1945 "Preface to New Edition" of that book, in which he addressed the many problems encountered by earlier readers in attempting to teach themselves, constitute the most useful material available for someone who is absolutely determined to go it alone. (Information on where to locate Alexander's writings can be found in "Suggestions for Further Reading" at the end of this book.)

It is unfortunate for the serious student that there are a few books which encourage readers to believe they can easily learn the Technique on their own in a few days, or weeks. These have usually been written by people with little personal experience of the Technique, and in at least one case, with *none* whatsoever — as extraordinary as that may seem!

The problem is not an entirely new one. Almost from the start of his teaching, Alexander was dogged by people bent on distorting and mis-representing his work. Sometimes it was for personal gain; more often because of ignorance. "If there is a crackpot within fifty miles," he once said, "he will find his way to me."

For an Alexander teacher, there is nothing more disheartening than getting a call from someone accouncing, "I've been practising the Alexander Technique, using ----'s book, and would like a refresher lesson." Sadly, we know what to expect: the pupil *has* made a change in his or her old habits, and inevitably for the worse. Typically, they have stiffened their bodies in an attempt to follow the written instructions, often alternating this new, harmful pattern with their previous bad habits. The teacher is thus confronted with a pupil with *two* distinct sets of misuse, their old one and their new "learned" one.

Teaching in these cases is doubly difficult, and extremely frustrating, for both pupil and teacher. What makes this particularly unfortunate is that these are usually highly motivated individuals who would normally make very rapid progress but who have been seriously misled into creating additional difficulties for themselves. Luckily, most readers of these books become so frustrated that they give up after a few days. The only lasting harm is the false impression of the Technique with which they are left.

The fact is that when expressed in purely verbal form without the corresponding kinesthetic information, Alexander's ideas are all too easily misunderstood and misapplied. That is what Alexander discovered when he first began to teach, before he developed a method of communicating with his hands. And that, of course, is why your teacher has had to go through such a long period of practical training.

When properly taught, the Technique encourages you to take responsibility for yourself as quickly as you are capable of doing so. It is almost certain that you will need a qualified teacher to get started, but his goal is always to enable you to become completely independent of him — to be able to make additional positive changes in yourself, *by* yourself.

In Chapter Three, we saw some of the ways in which the Alexander Technique has been applied to the relief of painful symptoms and the improvement of performance skills. These long-standing, "traditional", uses of the Technique are what it is best known for. In the final chapter, we'll explore some very interesting new applications that have been discovered in recent years.

Kevin, who is in his forties, is a principal lecturer in a College of Further Education in London.

"I consider myself to be just about the most unlikely candidate possible for getting involved with the Alexander Technique. A friend and colleague — we'd taught together for seven or eight years — was married to an Alexander teacher and both she and her husband had frequently tried to explain to me something about it. I'm a pretty practical down-to-earth person by nature and, frankly, it sounded to me like a lot of twaddle. I should say that I've always prided myself on being physically fit. I did a lot of weight training when I was younger and I love running — not just as a means to an end but for the great feelings I get out of it, both during and after. I swim a lot, too.

"Anyway, a few years ago, I suddenly started getting severe back pain — and I mean severe. It was really frightening — it came out of nowhere — no injury, nothing like that. For the first time I was taking time off work — weeks at a stretch — and whereas I'm not work-crazy, that's another thing I'd always prided myself on — turning up for my job and doing it properly. It's a terrific shock when you've always thought of yourself as really fit to be suddenly flat on your back with pain. And it was an even bigger shock when my doctor told me he couldn't do anything about it. His actual words were: 'It's your age: you're forty now. You can expect that sort of thing. You're just going to have to live with it.'

"It was at that stage in the proceedings that Nanette (my colleague) finally persuaded me to go to her husband for some Alexander Technique lessons. In fact, I didn't need much persuading — I was about ready to try anything — even wishing wells! As I've said, we were friends and they told me to come for a few weeks' worth of free lessons, the idea being that if I found them helpful I could then go to another teacher that I'd pay in the normal way.

"*I'll be honest with you, during that first lesson when Paul was talking and very lightly touching the back of my neck or shoulders — or my legs, feet, arms as I lay on the table — I was thinking to myself, in language a whole lot stronger than I'll use now, 'Thank goodness, I'm not actually paying for this nonsense . . .' I went back for the second lesson only because they were my friends and I was too embarrassed not to.*

"Anyway, it was after the second lesson that I started getting incredible muscular releases in my neck and across my shoulders. Nobody could have been more amazed than I was! I know a lot of people report very gradual changes with the Technique, but my own were pretty dramatic — I was out running again within a couple of weeks of that first lesson.

"I've continued with the Technique — not slavishly but with groups of lessons and the occasional workshop at fairly regular intervals. I've learnt a great deal and, ironically, I've had to admit that a lot of my problems were being created by precisely what I considered to be evidence of my 'fitness'. The muscles in my neck and shoulders and upper back, so highly developed by the weight training, were also 'locked' and inflexible, and were at the root of my back pain. I don't want to give the impression that the Alexander Technique has solved my problems by transforming me into a seven-stone weakling — God forbid — but I have been able to use it to release the tension in those areas.

"I now try to make up for my original cynicism by 'spreading the Alexander word' amongst my friends and colleagues, a spectacle which Nanette and Paul for some reason find amusing . . ."

6

RECENT DEVELOPMENTS

As we saw in Chapter Two, soon after Alexander made his original discoveries, and developed a specific method of teaching others, his work attracted the interest of two distinct groups. First, fellow performers quickly found in his Technique a remarkably effective way to improve their own performance skills. Second, members of the medical community — some of whom had earlier tried to help Alexander with his voice problem — were impressed by the beneficial effects his teaching had on pupils' health and began referring some of their patients to him.

As Alexander gained more experience, he began to realize that his teaching method could be used in many more ways than just these two applications of the Technique — applications which were described in some detail in Chapter Three. Sadly, Alexander died a few years before this happened to any great extent. But recently, with the increase in the number of trained teachers, many new and varied ways have been found to use the discoveries made by him nearly a century ago.

Rather than try to tell about all of them — which in any case couldn't be done in the space available here — I'll describe those applications which I've found to be of particular interest to my pupils, and to others with whom I've discussed the Technique.

First of all, they are frequently very curious about the relationship of the Technique to other ways of enhancing physical and mental well-being. This is to be expected; they have often tried, or considered, some of the methods themselves, or know others who have done so.

I also find that once pupils have experienced the beneficial effects of Alexander lessons, they are eager to find out if it could also help their friends and family. So quite often I am asked about its applications to the special requirements of pregnant women, children and the elderly.

In this chapter, I've drawn heavily on the knowledge and experience of colleagues of mine who, in addition to being qualified Alexander teachers, also have professional backgrounds in fields as diverse as chiropractic, massage therapy, childbirth education, osteopathy and the martial arts.

Yoga

A great many students and teachers of yoga have been helped by their study of the Alexander Technique. Indeed, several highly respected yoga instructors have found the Technique to be so valuable that they have undertaken the three years of training necessary to qualify as an Alexander teacher.

One of these is Chris Stevens, formerly Secretary General and Teacher Education Officer of the British Wheel of Yoga. He presently lives and teaches in Denmark. In his book *Yoga*, he writes:

"In my experience the Alexander Technique is the most effective way of learning to apply the basic principles of yoga. It teaches us how to observe ourselves in everyday life. We can then see how our harmful mental and physical habits affects everything we do. The Technique gives a practical way of stopping the habits and replacing them with consciously chosen natural ways of using the mind/body . . ."

I asked Mr. Stevens to say a bit more about his own experiences with yoga and the Alexander Technique.

"The yoga postures stopped being something I forced my body to do. Instead they became enjoyable experiments. However, the most important changes were in the way I approached my practices and *how* I carried them out rather than in what I did. Later I began to reread the yoga texts in the light of my Alexander experience and found interesting parallels between the two disciplines. For example, Patanjali is quite specific about what are the first practices in yoga. They are not postures but creative and sensible self control, a self observation that is free of all egoistical concern with 'results'. These first steps in yoga were exactly what I had found in my Alexander lessons.

"By learning how not to be bound up in results, I was able to attend to the *process* of my yoga practice. This helped me to learn more about myself and how my underlying attitudes, physical as well as mental, were profoundly affecting what I was doing. I further learnt that they affected the benefits (or lack of them) I got from my practices. In a word, I was becoming more conscious in a practical and useful way."

Ken Thompson has practiced yoga since 1955. He has collaborated on a number of books about yoga and is the present Teacher-Education Tutor, as well as the Chairman, of the Wheel of Yoga. At his centre in Ilford, Essex, Mr. Thompson teaches the Alexander Technique — he too is a qualified teacher — and all levels of yoga. He is particularly concerned with the inappropriate ways yoga has sometimes been practiced in the West:

"Many yoga students become so keen to achieve a certain position that they will give very little consideration as to whether the working integrity of the body is being maintained in the process.

"In padmassana (lotus) for instance, most people, once they see that the object of the exercise is to get both feet up onto opposite thighs, will make that their goal, and end-gain towards it. Some may find that padmassana comes easily to them almost from the first attempt, but for the vast majority it does not, so they struggle with it for months or years until they do it — then wonder why they have developed lower-back trouble or weak knees! What they don't realize is that their problem has been caused by forcing the legs into lotus position at the expense of the back. I am always reminding my students: 'If you don't do yourself any good, for heaven's sake don't do yourself any harm!'

"People often ask me how I relate the Alexander Technique to yoga. One thing that the two have in common is that yoga is not about acquiring knowledge but rather ridding oneself of ignorance: similarly, the Alexander Technique is not concerned with being right, but with avoiding going wrong.

"For me, the two systems complement each other. Yoga gives me a philosophy for living, while Alexander gives me the *means whereby* to do it — 24 hours a day!"

Physical Therapy

If you've ever had a serious injury, or been through a major operation, you probably have good reason to admire and respect the work of physical therapists. In many ways, they are the "unsung heroes" of modern medicine, as they struggle valiantly, often within severe time constraints, to help patients regain the physical abilities necessary to rebuild their lives.

Heather Kroll is an experienced physical therapist and Alexander Technique teacher who works at the Children's Hospital and Medical Center in Seattle, Washington. She has this to say about the Technique, and its relation to her hospital work:

"One of my primary jobs as a physical therapist is teaching. Whether I am working with an injured athlete or a brain damaged child, movement re-education is my focus. As a tool for movement re-education, the Alexander Technique is a great asset.

"Take the case of the injured athlete. Many sports related injuries are due to chronic over use, or chronic misuse. While ice, ultrasound, mobilization, soft tissue techniques and other modalities can help solve the acute problem, the athlete must change his or her movement habits to prevent the problem from recurring. The Alexander Technique is a tool which the athlete can take into the practice of sport and thereby improve performance and prevent future injury.

"In teaching back care and body mechanics, the Technique is a very effective way of helping people learn to observe themselves so that they actually know what they are doing to themselves that is harmful. With this knowledge, it is then possible to make lasting changes in movement habits.

"The Technique can also be applied to exercises. Most exercises are done with a specific end in mind — for example: increased strength, improved flexibility, or better posture. Exercises carried out with poor coordination reinforce that poor coordination. By using the Alexander Technique, both in teaching and doing exercises, poor movement habits, which interfere with results, are eliminated and the exercises then become much more effective.

"For myself, the Technique helps me to continually

improve my own skills. As a physiotherapist, I am able to move people easily and efficiently, so that at the end of the day I am neither hurt, nor overly tired."

The special problems associated with the management of scoliosis in adolescents and adults has been extensively studied by Deborah Caplan, a New York City physical therapist and teacher of the Alexander Technique. A study completed by her, under the supervision of an orthopedic surgeon, clearly showed that the Alexander Technique is a particularly effective way to help detect and eliminate the harmful postural habits characteristic of scoliosis.

Osteopathy

Unlike most medical doctors, osteopaths emphasize the diagnosis and treatment of disease by physical methods, resorting to drugs or surgery only as a last resort. Mervyn Waldman, D.O., is in private practice in London and, because he is also a qualified Alexander teacher, is able to discuss the contribution the Technique is beginning to make to the practice of osteopathy. This is what he has to say:

"From its inception, osteopathy — like the Alexander Technique — insisted on the importance of postural balance and good use. Indeed it is a great irony that J. M. Littlejohn, one of the most important founders of osteopathy, and F. M. Alexander lived within a half a mile of each other in London in the 1930's and 1940's, yet never met.

"Ensuring the minimum of postural strain on any part of the body, including internal viscera, has always been considered by osteopaths an essential preventive measure and an often vital therapeutic endeavour for sustained recovery. However, the means by which such measures were instituted, and instruction and advice given, were originally very crude in comparison to the work being undertaken by Alexander. Insufficient attention was paid to a number of interrelated factors: the strength of established and in-grained habit; the need to develop improved sensory aware-ness of the difference between good and faulty use of the self; the development of and capacity to consciously con-trol otherwise automatic and faulty response patterns ('sets') to a given stimulus; and finally the immense impor-tance of the head, neck, back relationship in determining the quality of use.

"Many injuries and illnesses are beyond nature's capa-city to repair unassisted by direct intervention. Of course, individual circumstances must always determine whether the emphasis should be placed on treatment or on lessons in the Technique. Generally speaking, however, I find that the insights gained from one system greatly assist in the application of the other.

"In my own practice, an appreciation of the intimate relationship between structure, use and function has en-couraged me to use the Technique to help some of the most infirm as well as those suffering from many of the constitutional diseases. In other cases, the use of osteo-pathic medicine had allowed a bed-ridden patient to be-come mobile and relatively free of disabling pain, thereby giving him an opportunity to improve his use with the Technique.

"My Alexander training has certainly been of great help to me in carrying out osteopathic procedures. These frequently pose demanding physical challenges and I find the Technique enables me to perform them in a way which minimizes stress and fatigue.

"Recently — and particularly in Britain — as osteo-paths have become familiar with Alexander's ideas and work, these have been readily admired and accepted by the profession for their sound rationale and practicality. And, when patients can be persuaded to adopt a concern for self-help and self-management, referrals are now being made to teachers of the Technique to supplement their treatment programme."

Chiropractic

For many North Americans, painful symptoms like backache, a stiff neck, or sore feet mean a visit to the family chiropractor. Despite what was originally, at best, only a grudging acceptance from the medical community, chiropractors have managed, in less than a century, to establish a secure position for themselves in our health care system. They have even begun to make significant inroads in Japan and several European countries.

Within the chiropractic community itself, a wide variety of approaches to health co-exist. I therefore decided it would be best to ask *two* chiropractors, both of whom are also qualified Alexander teachers, to say a little about how their Alexander training has influenced their treatment approach.

John M. Wynhausen, D.C., has a successful private practice in Lincoln, Nebraska. He notes that: "A well aligned spine is essential to spinal health. There are two basic ingredients to a well aligned spine. The first and most important is a habit of poise, or grace, along with free and easy movement in everyday life. The Alexander Technique of education helps the individual toward this end.

"The second ingredient is a spine free of vertebral subluxations — those minute dislocations within the spinal column. Scientific chiropractic adjustments supply this latter need.

"I have explored both these avenues of spinal health and found that one supports the other as elegantly as structure supports function. As a chiropractor and an Alexander teacher, I believe both of these ingredients are necessary for optimum health."

Donald L. Weed, D.C., is a neuromuscular reeducation specialist and a teacher at the Performance School in Seattle, Washington. This is what he has to say on the subject:

"While malcoordination only rarely causes a patient's condition, it can be harmful to one's overall health. One of the most frustrating experiences for a therapist is to work with a client, see him improve, and then watch him go back to his previous manner of movement which compromises some or all of the therapist's work.

"Too often, the patient's malcoordination in movement is the factor which prevents success in a treatment program. The movement work of F. M. Alexander is the best process I have ever seen for bringing about constructive changes in patient coordination. While not a therapy in itself, this educational process can give to the patient the tools needed to take a constructive role in the improvement of his or her condition.

"I firmly believe that the combination of what a trained health care professional can do for you with what you can do for yourself through Mr. Alexander's work is the best combination possible for improving your health."

Martial Arts

Many westerners have come to appreciate first hand the benefits to be found from the study of Karate, Aikido, Jujitsu and some of the other long-established martial art forms originating in the Orient. They offer much more than training in combat and self-defense — the kind of thing featured in so many violent Kung Fu movies. Indeed, many students are drawn to the martial arts primarily for their mental and spiritual rewards.

Pete Trimmer is a qualified Alexander teacher who

lives in Takoma Park, Maryland. He also holds a third degree Aikido black belt and this is what he has to say about one of the classic difficulties often encountered by the martial arts student, and how the Technique can help to overcome it:

"A concept that is one of the most basic and pervasive in all the martial arts is the importance of moving from the center and always staying centered. The very best martial artists develop this skill through years of experience and training. But many fail to learn how to do so. The Alexander Technique helps the martial artist to find his center and to consistently move from there, even in pressured situations.

"'Lower your center' is one of the most frequently used phrases in the martial arts. To do this, most people slump downwards, into their hips. This gives a false *feeling* of power and strength. In fact, they are really just producing a lot of harmful pressures throughout their body. This has two disastrous results: First, the energy going into producing this pressure is no longer available for combat. They can no longer attack and defend themselves with their full power. Second, these pressures severely decrease their mobility — their ability to respond swiftly and surely to their opponent's moves.

"The Alexander Technique helps the martial artist to become sensitive to his habits of movement. He learns to use whatever degree of tension is appropriate in a given situation and to release that tension when it is no longer useful. This means he is capable of quicker movement, stronger technique, greater flexibility and a better ability to respond to the unexpected."

Massage Therapy

The benefits, and the sheer *pleasure*, of a good massage

are appreciated by more and more people today. In addition to the more traditional Swedish style of working, there is a growing interest in alternative methods — Japanese Shiatsu, for example.

The old image of a brawny masseur or masseuse pounding away at the flesh and bones of the hapless victim has been replaced by one of a highly qualified massage therapist, using his or her skills to help promote the patient's overall health and well-being.

I asked Jane Kasdan Shelton, a Licensed Massage Therapist and teacher of the Alexander Technique in Atlanta, Georgia how she integrates the two methods of removing unwanted patterns of tension. She reports:

"For years I observed my massage clients get off the massage table, free or greatly eased of the complaints they arrived with, only to go back to their old, harmful habits of movement. It was just a matter of time before their problems returned. I decided to apply my training in the Alexander Technique to massage and I now begin each session with a short Alexander lesson. I find this produces changes that are dramatic and lasting."

"The use of the Alexander Technique with massage lets the client participate in removing tension. Each muscle receives an Alexander lesson: it learns to lengthen, spread out and fit in with the body as a whole, which allows the muscle to function easily. By employing the principles of the Technique to *my* body while giving a massage, I find my fingers no longer try to impose change, which always meets with resistance, but now function as a tool to help the client register unnecessary tension and then learn how to remove that tension.

"It is really an education in heightening awareness and control. A very rewarding experience for us both."

Pregnancy and Childbirth

It is well known — among women, at any rate — that the special *physical* demands of carrying an unborn child, and giving birth, are often as much of a challenge as the many other changes which come with motherhood. Doctors have long been aware of wide variations in women's ability to adapt to these demands. In their classic 1932 book, *Body Mechanics*, the authors — four orthopedic surgeons — stated:

> "Most of the gynaecological disabilities and long periods of weakness following some pregnancies can be explained on the basis that the compensation for long-standing faulty body mechanics has been broken by the burden of pregnancy and parturition, and when once broken, the badly used body is unable to regain its compensation and strength."

In *The Truth About Childbirth* (1937), Anthony Ludovici notes that with faulty use, and the accompanying poor body coordination, "we have a sufficient amount of mischief to impair not only the course of pregnancy but also and above all that of childbirth." Ludovici refers to the work of Alexander who, long before "natural childbirth" became fashionable, was teaching women how to stop interfering with the normal processes of gestation and delivery.

Over the years, many doctors and other health care workers have attested to the effectiveness of the Alexander Technique in helping with pregnancy and childbirth. Among them is Catherine Madden, a Certified Childbirth Educator, a mother, and a faculty member of the Performance School, a center for the study of the Alexander Technique in Seattle, Washington. Here is what she has to say on the subject:

"The Alexander Technique is the greatest 'comfort measure' that I could suggest to any woman who is pregnant. Book after book, class after class, describe specific ways for her to improve her posture and avoid back pain, tension and fatigue. But the aches and pains of pregnancy are frequently the result of poor use — often producing a strong back-and-down pressure in an attempt to compensate for the increasing weight of the child. This pressure pushes the abdomen forward, creating an unnatural hollow in the lower back. This excessive curvature, in turn, produces yet more harmful pressure on the hips, legs and feet.

"When a woman learns to use the Alexander Technique, she discovers that it is actually much easier to support her growing baby by letting her whole head and body move gently up. This restores her natural balance and flexibility. Not only does this often alleviate the back pains and pressures associated with pregnancy, but it also seems to aid in the function of all the internal organs. As pregnancy progresses these organs are pushed into a smaller and smaller space in order to make room for the growing fetus. Knowledge of the Alexander Technique helps a woman prevent any more compression of these organs than is necessary. I suspect — although I cannot yet document this — that women who know how to use the Technique have fewer kidney and bladder infections, less heartburn, and better blood circulation to the placenta and fetus.

"An example: One of the students in my childbirth education class called me to say her doctor told her she probably had a low-grade kidney infection. Yet she had no fever — in fact, the only symptom was persistent pain on her right side. As she walked into class that week, I saw that she was moving in a way that would indeed compress the organs on that side of her body. I suggested an Alexander lesson, and we found that the pain disappeared as she learned to release the downward pull that was responsible for the harmful pressure.

"The great advantage that the Alexander Technique gives a woman during labor and delivery is increased knowledge of her own body. Women who know the Technique have a process which helps them to use only those muscles which are necessary, making the birth process a whole lot easier and smoother."

Children

Alexander had always hoped that his discoveries would some day be applied to the *prevention* of mis-use, rather than the more time consuming task of undoing patterns that had become so deeply entrenched that they were causing pain or illness. He had a good deal of experience teaching children — they were usually brought to him by anxious parents who were worried about such things as their child's stammer, asthma or mal-coordination. The harmful posture and movement habits of these children were still comparatively weak and he found they could usually learn to regain their natural poise and balance in a very short period of time.

Like most other Alexander teachers, I have taught quite a number of children, usually after one or both of their parents have had at least a few lessons first. I never fail to be amazed at how easily most children learn the Technique and how quickly and spontaneously they apply their new knowledge to their daily activities. I am convinced that this has a lot to do with their ability to absorb non-verbal information directly, without filtering it through intellectual or judgmental faculties.

Over the years, there have been several experiments in introducing the Technique into the schoolroom. Most of these have taken place in England and one of them resulted in a book, *Choice of Habit*, by J. V. Fenton, a senior lecturer in Physical and Health Education at Wandsworth Training College of Teachers in London. Fenton describes the benefits that came from teaching the Technique at two schools of which he had been headmaster, and he urges that the study of posture and movement along the lines pioneered by Alexander be included in primary and secondary school curriculums.

Although the experiments conducted so far have been extremely successful, financial constraints have usually prevented them from moving beyond the exploratory stage. The result, tragically, is the all too often repetition of classroom scenes like the following:

> "A teacher calls her six and seven-year-olds to gather round her on the floor and listen to a story. Most sit cross-legged with their spines collapsed into a curve and their heads pulled back onto their necks as they look up at the teacher. One boy is kneeling close to the teacher, back beautifully aligned, head balancing on the top. 'Thomas, you are blocking the people behind you you', says the teacher, in a reproachful tone. 'Sit down so they can see the pictures.' The child sits down obediently and collapses like the others around him. The teacher does not see what has happened, does not see that she has required the child to go from a poised, balanced, alert position, to one that is cramped, and distorted. Knowing better than to protest, the child looks resigned."

This was recorded in a 1984 Master of Science thesis by Ann Matthews, a New York City teacher of the Alexander Technique. Her study of the application of the Technique in a classroom setting — by far the most thorough yet conducted — was based largely on her experiences teaching first and second grade pupils in a Rockland County, New York public school. Her work shows very clearly that young children can make dramatic improvements in their posture and movement patterns with only a small amount of very gentle guidance from an Alexander Teacher.

In his introduction to one of Alexander's books, John Dewey wrote:

> "(Alexander's) discovery would not have been made and the method or procedure perfected except by dealing with adults who were badly coordinated. But the method is not one of remedy; it is one of constructive education. *It's proper field of application is with the young, with the growing generation . . .*" (emphasis mine)

The work of Ms. Matthews, and the others who have brought the Technique into the classroom, confirms beyond a doubt the correctness of Dewey's belief. I will have more to say on this important subject in the Epilogue.

The Elderly

Many of Alexander's most famous pupils studied with him well into old age. For example, Professor John Dewey was 58 when he first met Alexander and he continued to have lessons from time to time until his death at the age of 93. George Bernard Shaw *started* taking lessons when he was in his eighties. Several of my own pupils have been people in their 70's and 80's.

Richard A. Brown is uniquely qualified to discuss the Technique as it relates to older people. He is an Alexander teacher with a busy practice in Boston, holds a Doctorate in Psychology, and for many years has researched the special problems of the elderly. He is also the author of several chapters of *Your Parent's Keeper: A Handbook of Psychiatric Care for The Elderly* by Jonathan Lieff, M.D. His description of the physiological changes that typically accompany the aging process makes for depressing reading:

"Studies have shown that between the ages of thirty and eighty, people lose on the average nearly half of their lung capacity. This is important because studies of health statistics have shown that those who lose the most lung capacity are likely to die significantly sooner.

"Other studies have shown, on the average, a two inch loss in height in men and women between the ages of 20 and 70. In addition to the shrinkage of the bones and soft tissues of the back, there is a shortening of stature due to increased curves in the spine. A characteristic mark of old age is the hunching forward of the upper back (dowager's hump). To compensate for this, there is a tendency to tilt the head back, exaggerating the curve in the neck. In some cases this can cause kinking in the arteries which supply blood to the head.

"The difficulty which some old people have in rising from a seated position is one sign of muscular weakness. Studies have shown progressive deterioration in muscle strength with increasing age, for example a 45% loss in grip strength between age 30 and 75."

That's the bad news. The good news is that while these signs of frailty are *statistically* more common in elderly people, they are *not* inevitable, or irreversible. As Dr. Brown reports:

"Numerous scientific studies have shown that some of the most serious physical problems associated with aging — shortness of breath, poor posture and co-ordination, and loss of strength — can be significantly reduced with the help of the Alexander Technique. Needless to say, any improvement in these areas makes a significant contribution to the quality of older people's lives, especially their ability to retain their independence."

I would like to add a non-scientific observation of my own to those of Dr. Brown: Alexander teachers themselves display a remarkable ability to live full, active lives well into old age. Many of those who were on Alexander's first training courses in the early 1930's are still, today, carrying a full teaching load.

****

Throughout this book, I have emphasized the practical benefits of the Technique. These are — quite rightly, I believe — what it has always been best known for. However, it would be remiss of me if I failed entirely to consider the broader philosophical concepts of Alexander's work. In the Epilogue, therefore, I will discuss some of these and consider their relevance for us in the closing years of the twentieth century.

Suzanne is a thirty year old urban planner who lives in Toronto, Canada.

"My husband had some back problems and was taking Alexander lessons. This got me thinking about having lessons myself. I suffered from migraine headaches. And I had also been having trouble with my neck. There seemed to be a real awkward knot in my neck that would get in the way whenever I turned my head. It was a problem when I was at work or driving. I couldn't easily turn my head to look in the rear view mirror or to see traffic behind me. I was getting pretty sick of it so I started taking lessons. By the second lesson, I had forgotten that my neck was a problem and within a few weeks, the migraines were a thing of the past. After these two problems went away, I started becoming interested in the whole process

itself, and what else I could do with it.

"I had a lot of tension in my hips and legs, which I think went back to my childhood. I was never very flexible in my legs. I began to realize that I didn't have to hold onto my legs so tightly — they weren't going to fall off! I just didn't need all that effort. Also, ever since I was a child, I was very tight between my shoulder blades. My gym instructors would always comment on it but I just assumed it was something I couldn't do anything about. I found that I was now able to release some of the tension there and my shoulder blades just weren't squeezed so tightly anymore.

"My job involves a lot of desk work. As an urban planner there is a lot of reading, writing, meetings to attend — and a lot of hours spent sitting in a chair. At times it's very stressful, trying to organize several things simultaneously. Frequently it all just piles up at once and there's no way you can spread it out. The Alexander Technique helped me to become aware of what I was doing with myself when that sort of thing happened, how I was actually making things worse by getting all tensed up. I find I can now just stop this tension from even getting started. Somehow the pressure at work doesn't bother me as much anymore and I think I probably do my job more efficiently. And the long hours sitting at my desk, which used to make my neck sore and my head ache, don't have that effect anymore. Actually, I feel ten years younger.

"I've noticed a big effect on my personality. I think, in fact I know, I used to be pretty uptight. That's really changed. I feel more comfortable around people and connect more easily with them. I'm kinder to myself, too. That's something I've definitely gotten from the lessons. The lessons made me see the importance of looking after myself, not in a selfish way, but just not ignoring myself. Also, the whole way a teacher works, the way he observes and thinks about things, has had a good effect on me. The

teacher is totally there for me and gives a clear, non-judgmental observation of what I'm doing to myself. I don't have to try to make a good impression or anything like that. I can just be myself and know that the teacher will help me in any way he can.

"I've always been very analytical. I tend to do something and then think a lot about it afterwards. But now I'm starting to realize that my thinking itself can change, even while I'm in the middle of an activity. There doesn't have to be a split between a physical action and a mental thought — they really are the same thing on two different levels. I find I can also avoid getting caught up in one particular train of thought. I can see more clearly what I'm doing with my thoughts, and, if it seems appropriate, I can make another choice.

"The more I use the Technique — at work, for example — the more I want to use it. This has certainly helped my career. Recently I was given a promotion and I'm sure it had a lot to do with my putting into practice what I've learned during my lessons.

"One more thing about the Technique: What I remember most about the first lesson was really being able to move, with the teacher's help, of course, with a grace and ease that I had never experienced before. But yet you're still a beginning student. It's a wonderful thing to experience. I think that taste of what is possible makes it easier to learn because you can see very clearly what you're after. It gives you something to look forward to."

EPILOGUE
Looking Ahead

Those who think that form is unimportant will miss the spirit as well, while those who cling to form lose the very spirit which they tried to preserve. Form and movement are the secrets of life, and the key to immortality.

Lama Govinda

As we have seen, some of the greatest thinkers of the twentieth century have keenly promoted F. M. Alexander's work and achievements. If we want a fuller understanding of his contribution, we have to ask ourselves what it was about the man, and the Technique he developed, that inspired their enthusiasm. Clearly it was *not* because an Australian actor overcame a voice problem, helped some of his colleagues with similar difficulties and then continued this on a broader scale in England. If that were the full extent of his work, it would undoubtedly have been viewed as useful and positive. But it would hardly call forth the public tributes that have been made by writers of acknowledged greatness, by distinguished philosophers and Nobel prize-winning scientists.

The fact is that Alexander was in the vanguard of those whose work and discoveries — in many different fields — have led us towards the possibility of healing the split in Western consciousness between "mind" and "body". Many of us can still remember a time when, in the popular mind, "psychosomatic", with its literal Greek meaning of mind-body, meant "imaginary", "unreal", even "hypo-chondrichal". And for some people, that misapprehension persists.

It often comes as a shock to realize the extent to which our everyday ways of thinking spring from concepts that have long since been discarded by the scientific community. When we examine more closely attitudes and beliefs that we consider to be self-evident, obvious, just a matter of "common sense", we are often amazed to discover that they have been unconsciously shaped by temporary cultural fashions or outdated theories. For the irony — and the tragedy — is that it takes a very long time for the most advanced scientific thoughts to filter down to our general awareness.

In the present century in particular, the gap this has created between our knowledge of ourselves, and our knowledge of the world around us, has widened to the danger point. Only recently are we beginning, at the *individual* level, to challenge the destructive mind-body division fostered by the mechanistic view of the world, and the universe, which derived from classic Newtonian physics. Yet this view has long since been superseded in the scientific community by the discoveries of Albert Einstein and his successors. The "new" physics, which is having so much impact on our present thinking, was, in fact, largely in place early in this century.

So too were the foundations of Alexander's work. Alexander did not set out to make a profound philosophical contribution to twentieth century thought. On the contrary, as we have already seen, he was a man with a problem to which he sought a practical answer. However, in the long and patient process of solving that problem, he made discoveries about human behavior that have enormous and far reaching implications.

Because we human beings are intelligent, self-aware creatures, we naturally try to economize energy, both physical and mental, in carrying out the more routine aspects of our lives. In other words, we develop habits. Many of these habits are immensely useful, for they free our minds to explore more interesting terrain. To take a mundane example, we are perfectly able to have an interesting conversation while we sit peeling potatoes!

However, as with so many other things, habits are excellent servants but appalling masters. Without realizing it, we can easily develop ones that are harmful, precisely because, by definition, we do not pay attention to them. There exists no *automatic* self-correcting mechanism.

Of course we eventually notice the unfortunate results of these habits, results that we are frequently encouraged to blame on things like "stress", or badly designed furniture, or a disease visited upon us by some unknown agency. But by blaming something outside ourselves, we often preclude the possibility of self-examination and discovery of the root cause of the difficulty.

Alexander found that it was possible to re-direct our thinking so as to become aware of precisely what *we* are doing to ourselves, to identify what is not helpful, and then to stop doing it. Perhaps even more important, he was able to develop a *technique*, a specific method, for enabling us to do this.

It was not just a question of ideas and insights – though it certainly was that, too. His genius lay in developing a method for translating those insights into practical benefits. Moreover, it was a technique which he could train others to teach, so that those benefits could continue to be passed on after his death.

The importance of this link joining Alexander's *ideas*, on the one hand, with the verifiable physical *results* of his work, on the other, was emphasized by John Dewey when he wrote:

"It is one thing to teach the need of a return

to the individual man as the ultimate agency in whatever mankind and society collectively can accomplish. It is another thing to discover the *concrete procedure* by which this greatest of all tasks can be executed. *And this indispensable thing is exactly what Mr. Alexander has accomplished."* (emphasis mine)

The Alexander Technique is not a philosophy, or a religion, or a system of morality. However, it can be an enormously useful catalyst to our understanding in these areas, if we choose to use it in that way. By enhancing our self awareness, by increasing our ability to distinguish between what is natural and what is merely habitual, it can hardly fail to increase our power of understanding in the broadest terms.

Let me be clear: I am certainly not making extravagant claims that the Technique is some kind of abstract elixir that will make geniuses of the dull witted. What I do maintain — and this brings us back to the interconnectedness of mind and body — is that the objective self-examination and self awareness it fosters at the physical level has an inevitable carry over to the mental. And the physical release and the unlocking which it encourages can profoundly influence the way pupils think about themselves and the world around them.

John Nicholls, an experienced English teacher and director of an Alexander teacher training course in Australia, makes much this same point:

"In the ordinary way of things, when people have private Alexander lessons, the Technique really is just a tool . . . it does not contain within itself an explicit philosophy, religion, set of ethics, morality or anything like that. You can then use it to become better at whatever you choose to become better at. If you wish to lead a more principled or moral life according to some standards that you have to set yourself, it will almost certainly help you to do that. But — if we took as an example someone who is a burglar — it is perfectly true to say that if he wanted to become more effective at robbing other people he would become much more effective at it . . .

"Yet . . . the experience of some individuals who've gone very deeply into the Technique suggests that it may help in the construction of a *personal* morality out of one's own experience... the Alexander Technique may bring out a moral guide inherent in the *individual*, not in the Technique itself."

It is worth noting that while the majority of pupils still stress the physical benefits of the Technique, a growing number have felt that there were significant spiritual connotations to their experience with Alexander's work.

Aldous Huxley was one of the most prominent of these. Writing in the 1940s, he stated in no uncertain terms his conviction that the mental and spiritual aspects of the Technique are at least as important as the more obvious physical ones:

"Up to the present time, only two solutions have been discovered to the problem of bridging the gap between idealistic theory and actual practice. The first, which is very ancient, is the mystic's technique of transcending personality in a progressive awareness of ultimate reality. The second, which is very recent, was discovered some 50 years ago by F. M. Alexander and may be described as a technique for the proper use of the self, a method for the creative conscious control of the whole psychophysical organism . . . .

"(As a result of Alexander's discoveries) it
is now possible to conceive of a totally new type
of education affecting the entire range of human
activity, from the physiological, through the intellectual, moral, and practical, to the spiritual — an
education which, by teaching the proper use of
the self, would preserve children and adults from
most of the diseases and evil habits that now
afflict them."

Other pupils have come to similar conclusions. It is interesting, for example, how many nuns, priests, ministers
and rabbis take Alexander lessons. One of my pupils, a
Catholic nun, made this observation:

"The Technique has shown me a whole spirituality built around body awareness. For the first
time, I realize that when I get in touch with my
own body, I have a much better chance of getting
deeply in touch with my innermost self, which is
a composite of body, mind and spirit."

Working within a quite different spiritual framework,
David, a young Tai Chi master from California, has this to
say about his experience with the Technique:

"I have a particular interest in the Alexander
Technique: I find that it can enhance Kundalini
energy. This is an expression of dormant energy
at the base of the spine that is released and moved
upward through the body if the conditions are
correct. Working with that energy is really taking
your body's physical energy and transmuting it to
a spiritual plane."

Gordon, a middle aged minister of a large Protestant church in Lincoln, Nebraska, made the following comments on the Technique:

"Before I came to the Alexander Technique, I realized the importance of the mental-spiritual connection. But now I see more clearly than I ever have before that this mentality and spirituality had sure better happen to me at the physical level too, or I'll be stuck somewhere I don't want to be. The inner world and the outer world have to match in some kind of participatory harmony.

"One of the wounds, the brokennesses, of churches today is that they have been cutting off the human body below the neck. The denial, the guilt, the negation of "flesh and body" is all part of this. I believe the quality of church teachings in the future is going to depend on its willingness to bring the mind and body back together in harmony."

****

Perhaps the best way to appreciate the wider significance of Alexander's work is to consider a few of the ways in which a greater awareness of the principles of the Technique would affect our lives on a scale beyond the personal.

Let us look first at a subject which is a prime concern to all of us: the development of our children.

As we saw in the last chapter, Alexander himself always emphasized that the Technique really belongs in the schools because it is much more efficient to work with children, in whom destructive habits were not so deeply ingrained, than with adults.

One huge advantage of a movement in that direction would be that when those children in turn became parents, with an understanding of the dynamics of posture, they would be far less likely to force their own children to stand, walk or even toilet train before they were ready to embark on these at their own pace. With even a little background in the Technique, they would easily spot the stress patterns — the rigid holding of body and limbs, the restricted breathing, and the neck tension — that *always* accompany prematurely encouraged activities. Every child has his own internal program for embarking on these and if he is pushed beyond that, his coordination will inevitably suffer — often for the rest of his life.

I witnessed a striking example of this in my own teaching. Some years ago, a middle aged woman came to me for a series of lessons. She had a pronounced pattern of holding her elbows out to the side, while hunching up her shoulders. It was a pattern that was always strongest when she began to walk. We had made a lot of progress in other areas, for instance with the migraines and stiff neck she had originally complained of, but this arm/shoulder pattern seemed quite intractable. She always looked as if she were *afraid* of walking.

I finally asked her to bring any early childhood photos she might have and she found one taken when she was just one year old. There she was, walking towards the camera, an expression of terror on her face — and her arms and shoulders in *precisely* the same awkward pattern evidenced over half a century later! Her parents were always pushing her into doing things as early as possible, and preferably in advance of the other children in her age group — whether it was walking, playing the piano or graduating from high school.

The pattern never completely disappeared. But, after seeing it so clearly displayed in the photograph, and understanding why it had been produced, she was eventually able to let go of it to a very large extent. Even more important, her walking, and indeed all her movements, took on a far more alive and confident quality.

In addition to being sensitive to their children's stress patterns, parents educated in the Technique would also be far less likely to pass bad habit patterns on to their children. Children unconsciously copy the postural and movement patterns of the people around them, especially those of their parents, the adults they are most exposed to in infancy. When parents hold, or even touch, their children, they are, in effect, giving them something like an Alexander Technique lesson. Unfortunately, if the parent's own use is bad, that is what will be communicated to the child.

This can have very serious long-term consequences. All too often, patterns responsible for symptoms like backache, poor vision, and migraines in the mother or father are inadvertently transferred to their offspring and produce in them almost identical symptoms, years — or even decades — later.

But just as bad use can easily be transferred from one generation to the next, so too can good use. You probably can think of families whose members all seem to possess a natural grace, an ease and economy of movement. This is the norm in many so-called "primitive" cultures and, with the kind of re-education which the Alexander Technique provides, there is no reason at all why this could not become true of our own society too.

With an understanding of Alexander's discoveries, school teachers could play a major role in spotting early signs of mis-use in their young pupils. Particularly in the early grades of school, small changes and gentle suggestions can make a big difference. Putting a little less pressure on a child who is learning to write, for example, can frequently help eliminate much of the unnecessary tension in face, arms, hands — in the whole body, really — that is so often to be seen when young children are learning to push a pen across a page.

It's a tragic irony that this sort of stressful reaction is

still often interpreted as a sign that the child is "making an effort", and is actually rewarded with praise, or good marks. This of course simply reinforces the pattern and makes it even more likely that the same kind of harmful tension will accompany the child's acquisition of any new skill.

The study by Ann Matthews, mentioned in the last chapter, shows that classroom teachers who are provided with even brief exposure to the Technique, become very sensitive to effects of this kind. They quickly find that when their pupils are encouraged to carry out their activities with less unnecessary physical effort, they are far more likely to do them well — and with interest and enthusiasm.

School designers and administrators, too, could make a major contribution to their pupils' health and well being by paying closer attention to environmental factors — being alert, for instance to the harm done by seating small children of differing sizes in non-adjustable desks for hours at a time. A child hunched over a desk that doesn't fit him, peering forward to see the blackboard, can easily develop the habit of tightening his neck to retract his head — a pattern that ultimately can interfere with his performance for the rest of his life. It is no coincidence that mis-use in children usually becomes noticeable within a year or two of attending school.

There are many other ways in which the Alexander Technique can make important contributions to our childrens' development and, of course, ultimately to the entire population. And the benefits would not be limited to the physical, as important as those would be. Children who are free of unnecessary tension in their bodies, whose natural flexibility and coordination have not been smothered, will be far better able to learn and to develop the vast array of skills needed to function effectively in the adult world.

Let's turn now to a somewhat different subject. By

providing us with the sensitivity to know what is going on with ourselves, *and* the ability to change what we don't like, the Technique can do much to help alleviate the feeling of alienation and powerlessness which has become so prevalent in Western societies. Pupils frequently comment on the sense of empowerment they get from being able to successfully apply what they learn in lessons to challenging situations. They are not speaking of power over *others*, but of power to determine the direction their own lives will take. Often for the first time in years, they have a sense of being in control of their own destiny. They feel – and look – more alive and, significantly, have a sense of being more "connected" to others, and to the world around them.

We sometimes tend to be a bit like the cameraman who surveys objects and people around him, but who forgets to turn the camera on himself. The Alexander Technique brings us back to ourselves, not in a narcissistic way, but in a constructive one. We are then far less likely to allow *outside* pressures – from our work, or from family disputes, for example – to produce unnecessary tension *inside* us. This will not of course make our problems just disappear. But it does enable us, individually and collectively, to deal with them in a more effective manner, and with far less harm to ourselves.

Among other things, this increased sensitivity to ourselves would also bring with it a much greater appreciation of the importance touch can play in our lives. It is in fact an *extremely* powerful medium, though in the West it often tends to be relegated to a relatively few areas, like sex, child-parent contact and our relationship to pets. An enhanced understanding of the role of touch – and other non-verbal forms of communication – would certainly reduce the number of confusing "double messages" we so often encounter: a person's words saying one thing, his facial expression or body language another, often the exact opposite. This is particularly harmful for small children; contradictory messages from parents and other adults produce the classic "double bind" which can so easily lead to neurosis in the vulnerable young recipient.

With a greater understanding of Alexander's work, our present approach to physical training would certainly undergo a major transformation. At the very least, it would begin to shift away from today's narrow focus, with its heavy emphasis on quantity, not quality, of movement. As we saw in Chapter One, there is a growing awareness that something has gone terribly wrong with our approach to fitness, and some remedial changes are already being made to lessen a few of the more obvious dangers.

The principles Alexander discovered give us a constructive framework within which we can move beyond merely patching up the present system. It provides us with the means to do much more than just avoid injuries — important though that is. It can show us how to use our bodies, and ourselves, in ways that expand our physical and mental capacities and help promote our overall well being.

Drawing on his own experience, George Leonard, the author of *The Ultimate Athlete*, gives us a vision of what this kind of truly *restorative* approach to physical fitness could accomplish:

> "I've learned that a hard, unyielding body is not necessarily a strong body, and that to reveal emotions is not to be weak. I've seen how the constricted musculature that goes with a rigid, guarded attitude toward life actually impedes the flow of life energy, how it blocks joy and empathy, how it helps create efficient monsters who can dominate nature and other people, and who may yet destroy humankind on this planet. Most important, I've learned that all this can be changed, turned around, not just for me, but for

everybody, male and female, young and old, active and sedentary, skinny and fat."

The connection Leonard draws between the way we use ourselves and our future as a species is one which Alexander stressed over and over in his own writings. A greater appreciation of his work would help us to understand why, in so many social, political and economic spheres, our worthy goals are often frustrated — why, all too frequently, "the road to hell" really *is* paved with good intentions.

Alexander's work places a great deal of emphasis on the *way* a change is made — the *process* of change. Teachers know, and pupils quickly learn, that if this process is faulty, the goal will inevitably be frustrated.

This principle, so clearly evident at an individual level, also holds true for society as a whole. All too often, attempts by governments and other organizations to solve a problem fail miserably and create a host of new difficulties as well. Classic examples of this, familiar to Americans and many Europeans, are the post-war programs designed to provide housing for low income families. This was a highly worthwhile goal by any standards.

But *how* was it done? In the United States, by the creation of massive housing "projects"; in Great Britain and Europe, by their equivalent "tower blocks". With few exceptions, these "solutions" to the housing crisis were ugly, badly designed, and shoddily built. Often they destroyed older, viable neighborhoods with what soon became costly, high-rise, crime-infested slums. Some are now actually being demolished — not because the buildings are physically worn out, but because they have proved to be, quite literally, uninhabitable by human beings.

It would be ludicrous to suggest that if politicians and urban planners were given a few Alexander lessons they would be able to avoid such tragic mistakes in the future. But I do think that if they had a clearer understanding of the fact that the manner in which a plan is carried out is at least as important as the goal of the plan — the kind of understanding that a student of the Alexander Technique gains in a very concrete and personal way — they would be less likely to make the kinds of mistakes that so often sabotage the very best of intentions.

John Dewey made much the same point when he observed, "if our habitual judgements of ourselves are warped because they are based on vitiated sense material — as they must be if our habits of managing ourselves are already wrong — then the more complex the social conditions under which they live, the more disastrous must be the outcome."

Dewey's fear of the terrible consequences that could befall mankind in an increasingly complex world — *and* his belief that there is a way of avoiding catastrophe — are clearly evident in this remarkable pair of statements, made over a decade before the appearance of the Atom Bomb:

> "In the present state of the world it is evident that the control we have gained of physical energies, heat, light, electricity, etc., without having first secured control of our use of ourselves, is a perilous affair. Without (this) our use of other things is blind; it may lead to anything."

> "If there can be developed a technique which will enable individuals to secure the right use of themselves, then the factor on which depends the final use of all other forms of energy will be brought under control. Mr. Alexander has evolved this technique."

****

The late nineteenth and early twentieth century saw huge leaps forward in both human understanding and human technology. It was the era of Sigmund Freud, Albert Einstein, the Wright brothers, and a host of others who transformed our lives with long distance communications, motion pictures, the internal combustion engine, and so on.

Walter Carrington is an Alexander teacher and scholar who trained with Alexander in the 1930s and who is currently Director of the Constructive Teaching Centre in London, England – a long-established training course for Alexander teachers. He had this to say on Alexander's position in the historical context:

"I consider that Alexander's work is probably one of the most underrated achievements of the 20th century. I think it is surprising how relatively unknown and unrecognized it is, because I am convinced that it will prove to be as important to humanity as the work of Newton, of Einstein and particularly of Darwin."

This was written in 1969. Since then Alexander's work has achieved a much greater degree of recognition in medical and scientific circles.

Indeed, no less a figure than Nikolass Tinbergen, in his acceptance speech for the 1973 Nobel Prize for Medicine, said of Alexander's discoveries: "This story of perceptiveness, of intelligence and of persistence, shown by a man without medical training, is one of the true epics of medical research and practice."

It would certainly seem that Mr. Carrington's prediction about the future assessment of Alexander's contribution is now well on its way to being validated.

SUGGESTIONS FOR FURTHER READING

Reading about the Alexander Technique can never substitute for direct experience. And it is entirely possible to derive full benefits from lessons in the Technique without doing any reading at all on the subject. Indeed, some teachers themselves attach very little importance to what might be termed the "philosophical", or "intellectual" aspects of Alexander's work.

However, I have found that at some point many pupils do want to explore these areas. Most often, their interest develops *after* they have had lessons and made some important changes in themselves. It is at this point that they frequently want to learn more about a set of ideas which is having such a powerful effect on their lives.

In the present volume, I have of necessity omitted many details about the history and development of the Technique. Space limitations have also prevented me from doing full justice to many of the important concepts developed by Alexander and his followers.

Fortunately, other writers have covered that territory in several excellent studies. Among these are:

Body Awareness in Action by Frank Pierce Jones (New York: Schoken, 1976)
    One of the best books available on the development of the Technique. The author provides a clearly written overview of Alexander's work and describes the early experimental studies on the Technique he conducted at Tufts University.

Body Learning by Michael Gelb (New York: Delilah Books, 1981)
    A well-written, straightforward introduction to Alexander's ideas; contains many excellent photographs.

The Alexander Technique by Wilfred Barlow, M.D. (New York: Alfred Knopf, 1976)

Although this book is primarily concerned with the medical aspects of the Technique, Dr. Barlow also devotes considerable attention to the all-important link between our use and our ability to function effectively.

F. Matthias Alexander — The Man and His Work by Lulie Westfeldt (Westport, Connecticut: Associated Booksellers, 1964; re-issued in 1986 by Centerline Press)

The author provides a personal account of her lessons with Alexander and her experiences as a student in his first teacher training course in London. The book also includes a good description of Alexander's basic discoveries.

For those who want a more complete understanding of F. M. Alexander's work, there is no better source than his own writings. He wrote four books between 1910 and 1941: *Man's Supreme Inheritance, Constructive Conscious Control, The Use of The Self,* and *The Universal Constant in Living.* Be forewarned, however, that his leisurely writing style is not always easy going for the modern reader. (An exception is *The Use of The Self* which is much more tightly written.) All of Alexander's books are being re-issued in paperback by Centerline Press (address below).

An excellent alternative to tackling Alexander's books directly is provided by *The Resurrection of The Body — The Essential Writings of F. Matthias Alexander*, edited by Edward Maisel (New York: Delta Books, 1969, re-issued in 1986 by Shambhala). This is a skillfully produced volume combining some of Alexander's own writings, John Dewey's prefaces to his first three books, and an insightful overview of the Technique by Maisel himself.

Parents, teachers and others concerned with child development will find the thesis by Ann Matthews (cited in Chapter Six and in the Epilogue) an invaluable source of information. It is entitled "Implications for Education in the Work of F. M. Alexander: An Exploratory Project in a Public School Classroom" and is available by mail from the Institute for Research, Development and Education in the Alexander Technique, 74 MacDougal Street, New York, N.Y. 10012. The cost is $15 in the U.S. and Canada; $20 overseas.

Video tapes (on both North American and European VHS-format) of Alexander Technique teaching by master teachers are available from Fyncot Films, F. M. Alexander Films, The Alexander Technique Training Centre, and from Centerline Press (addresses below). These are particularly valuable for those with a special interest in human movement potential — doctors, chiropractors, athletic coaches, performance teachers, physical and occupational therapists etc.

Although not about the Technique, *The Art of Seeing* by Aldous Huxley (Seattle: Montana Books, 1975; re-issue of original 1942 publication) is well worth reading for anyone concerned with vision re-education, for themselves and, particularly, for their children. Huxley describes the work of Dr. William Bates, an American ophthalmologist whose pioneering work in this field bears many striking parallels to that of Alexander.

Tufts University, in co-operation with the Alexander Technique Association of New England, has established an archival collection of original materials relating to F. M. Alexander and the Alexander Technique, including the detailed results of numerous scientific investigations. For more information, write to the Curator, The Frank Pierce Jones Collection, Wessel Library, Tufts University, Medford, Massachusetts 02155.

Finally, for those who would like to learn about current developments in the study and practice of the Alexander Technique, the Alexander community's two journals are an excellent source of information:

Direction — A Journal of The Alexander Technique
c/o Fyncot Films
P.O. Box 27075
Seattle, Washington 98125
USA
(for North American subscribers)

or

c/o Fyncot Films
4-150 Holt Avenue
Cremorne, N.S.W. 2090
AUSTRALIA
(for Australian/N.Z. subscribers)

or

Fyncot Films
c/o Shirley Crawford
The Old School House
Ide Hill
Sevenoaks, Kent TN146 JT
ENGLAND
(for British and European subscribers)

The Alexander Journal
10 London House
266 Fulham Road
Londond SW10 9EL
ENGLAND

The Alexander Review
c/o Centerline Press
Suite 325
2005 Palo Verde Avenue
Long Beach, California 90815
USA

The Alexander Technique Training Centre
Attention: Jorgen Haahr
King Edward VI College
Fore Street
Totness, Devon TQ9 5RP
ENGLAND

F. M. Alexander Films
P.O. Box 408
Ojai, California 93023
USA
(805) 646-8902

PROFESSIONAL SOCIETIES
OF TEACHERS OF THE ALEXANDER TECHNIQUE

Society of Teaching of the Alexander
   Technique (STAT)
10 London House
266 Fulham Road
London, England SW10 9EL
Tel: 351-0828

American Guild of Teachers of the Alexander
   Technique (AGTAT)
931 Elizabeth Street
San Francisco, California 94114
Tel: (415) 282-8967

and

1913 Thayer Avenue
Los Angeles, California 90025
Tel: (213) 470-2672

North American Society of Teachers of the
   Alexander Technique (NASTAT)
P.O. Box 148026
Chicago, Illinois 60614-8026
Tel: (312) 472-2404

(STAT membership is worldwide; most North American teachers are members of AGTAT or NASTAT, so if you live in the United States or Canada, it would be best to send for *both* lists. Please include a stamped, self-addressed, envelope if possible.)

The following national societies are affiliated with STAT:

AUSTRALIA
Australian Society of Teachers of the Alexander
    Technique
P.O. Box 529
Milton's Point, N.S.W.
Tel: (02) 92.4499 (Mon-Fri, 9:30 AM to 1:30 PM)

CANADA
Canadian Society of Teachers of the F. M. Alexander
    Technique
P.O. Box 744
Station P
Toronto, Ontario M5S 2Z1
Canada

DENMARK
Danish Society of Teachers of the Alexander Technique
Solsmarkvej 20
8240 Risskov, Denmark
Tel: 06-174560

GERMANY
The Society of Teachers of the Alexander Technique
Postfach 5312
7800 Freiburg, West Germany

ISRAEL
Haifa School of the Alexander Technique
7 Hanadin Avenue
Haifa, Israel
Tel: 04-242-090

SWITZERLAND
Schweizerischer Verband der Lehrer der
   F. M. Alexander-Technik
Grendelweg 4
Ch — 4432 Lampenberg
Switzerland

RESIDENTIAL COURSES

A worldwide listing of residential courses in the Alexander Technique may be obtained from:

Alexander Technique Residential Workshops
Michael Frederick, Director
P.O. Box 408
Ojai, California 93023
USA
(805) 646-8902

A NOTE TO THE READER

My purpose in writing this book has been, quite simply, to help make F. Matthias Alexander's discoveries known to as many people as possible, for I am convinced that his work will prove to be of immense importance to us all as we face the unique challenges and opportunities of the late twentieth century. The problem in doing this — as anyone who has had experience with the Alexander Technique can testify — is that neither the process, nor its benefits, can be adequately described with words.

Notwithstanding this limitation, I have elected to continue writing on the subject and would therefore be grateful for your comments, and your suggestions for more effective ways to bridge the gap between descriptions of the Technique, on the one hand, and firsthand knowledge of it, on the other. I am also compiling a collection of pupils' experiences with the Technique, so I am particularly interested in hearing from readers who have gone on to take Alexander lessons themselves.

In addition to writing, I spend a good deal of my time teaching and I welcome inquiries from prospective pupils interested in organizing an Alexander Technique workshop in their community.

Robert M. Rickover
P.O. Box 27075
Seattle, Washington 98125
USA

Metamorphous Press

METAMORPHOUS PRESS is a publisher and distributor of books and other media providing resources for personal growth and positive changes. MPI publishes and distributes leading edge ideas that help people strengthen their unique talents and discover that we all create our own realities.

Many of our titles have centered around NeuroLinguistic Programming (NLP). NLP is an exciting, practical and powerful model of human behavior and communication that has been able to connect observable patterns of behavior and communication to the processes that underlie them.

METAMORPHOUS PRESS provides selections in many subject areas such as communication, health and fitness, education, business and sales, therapy, selections for young persons, and other subjects of general and specific interest. Our products are available in fine bookstores around the world. Among our Distributors for North America are:

Bookpeople   The Distributors
New Leaf Distributors   Inland Book Co.
Pacific Pipeline   Starlite Distributors

For those of you overseas, we are distributed by:
Airlift (UK, Western Europe)
Bewitched Books (Victoria, Australia)

New selections are added regularly and the availability and prices change so ask for a current catalog or to be put on our mailing list. If you have difficulty finding our products in your favorite store or if you prefer to order by mail we will be happy to make our books and other products available to you directly.

YOUR INVOLVEMENT WITH WHAT WE DO AND YOUR INTEREST IS ALWAYS WELCOME — please write to us at:

Metamorphous Press, Inc.
3249 N.W. 29th Avenue
P.O. Box 10616
Portland, Oregon 97210
(503) 228-4972